Zoonoses

8

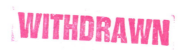

Zoonoses

Martin Shakespeare

BPharm, MRPharmS, Dip AgVet, Dip CP(DES), RNR

Community Pharmacy Manager
York, UK

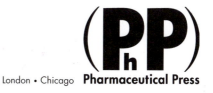

London • Chicago **Pharmaceutical Press**

Published by the Pharmaceutical Press
Publications division of the Royal Pharmaceutical Society of Great Britain

1 Lambeth High Street, London SE1 7JN, UK
100 South Atkinson Road, Suite 206, Grayslake, IL 60030-7820, USA

© Pharmaceutical Press 2002

First published 2002

Text design by Barker/Hilsdon, Lyme Regis, Dorset
Typeset by Photoprint, Torquay, Devon
Printed in Great Britain by TJ International, Padstow, Cornwall

ISBN 0 85369 480 X

A catalogue record for this book is available from the British Library

Contents

The colour plate section is between pages 114 and 115.

Preface

This book is aimed at trained and trainee healthcare professionals. The intention is to provide, in a compact format, an introduction and easily accessible reference for the more commonly encountered zoonotic diseases. This volume also aims to increase awareness and understanding of zoonoses amongst healthcare professionals, not only within the context of domestic disease, but also in the wider world. Healthcare and healthcare problems become more international every day, and with the massive increase in numbers of people travelling from place to place for business or pleasure, it is increasingly necessary for us to widen our horizons, so as to be able to respond appropriately to patient needs.

It is hoped that readers will gain some understanding of the constant challenge that these diseases present to healthcare and our society, and the ways in which these conditions are so important in our history, infrastructure and lives.

As an author I would be delighted if all my readers consume the whole volume at one sitting; however, the case studies and chapters of diseases related to particular risk groups and animal genera are meant for use as a reference for occasional use. Several of the chapters are meant to stand alone, and wherever possible suitable references have been given. These are included not only to show the source material used for the text; many of them offer further reading or detail concerning the conditions covered.

There is an emphasis on those zoonoses which are considered to be significant, established or emerging in the UK, and that are likely to present in domestic healthcare settings in the sections on companion and domestic animals. However for some sections of the volume, conditions or disease states have been included which have a worldwide significance, not only for completeness, but also for information and educational purposes.

Chapter 6, designated Pandora's Box, aims to dispel some of the mythology surrounding the more emotive and dramatic zoonoses found elsewhere in the world, especially those where media reporting may be too dramatic for more scientific tastes.

I hope that readers will find this book as rewarding to read as I found it challenging and interesting to write.

Martin Shakespeare
February 2002

Acknowledgements

The material on which this book is based was researched after a series of chance remarks, idle words and rash promises. My thanks go primarily to my wife, Josephine Sheppard, for tolerating and encouraging its lonely creation; also to Andrew Cairns (Chairman of the Veterinary Group of the Royal Pharmaceutical Society) and Liz Griffiths (Secretary of the same group) for their help and support in exploring and developing the project on which this volume is based. My thanks also go to my staff, who have put up with my babblings about these conditions for 'too long'.

This book has had about the gestational time of an elephant, so I feel the words of Rudyard Kipling are appropriate. They form the basis upon which I have always explored and learnt anything. I commend them to you.

> I keep six honest serving-men
> (They taught me all I knew);
> Their names are What and Why and When
> And How and Where and Who.
>
> *The Elephant's Child* by Rudyard Kipling

About the author

Martin Shakespeare graduated in 1980 with a Bachelor of Pharmacy degree from the London School of Pharmacy, University of London, and went on to undertake his preregistration year at St Bartholomew's Hospital, London. After registration he continued his studies by undertaking the Diploma in Crop Protection at Harper Adams Agricultural College, Shropshire.

Whilst working in community pharmacy, he completed the Diploma in Agricultural and Veterinary Pharmacy in 1986. His subsequent career was very varied, and it was not until 1996 that he re-entered the field of agricultural and veterinary pharmacy. A long-standing interest in zoonoses led to Martin being invited to make a presentation at the British Pharmaceutical Conference in 1999. The writing of an education package for the Scottish Centre for Post Qualification Pharmaceutical Education on zoonoses for pharmacists followed in early 2000, with the material being developed and expanded to produce the present volume.

1

Introduction to zoonoses

The basic definition

In the study of any scientific subject it is important that the terms used are understood from the outset. Zoonoses are no exception. The first question has to be: what is a zoonosis? The best agreed definition is that developed and used by the World Health Organization. This defines a zoonosis as:

> Those diseases and infections which are naturally transmitted between vertebrate animals and man.

As with many definitions, there are some conditions that are considered to be zoonoses, but which lie outside the strict application of the term. For example, *Ciguatera* and the related complex of shellfish poisonings are the result of ingested toxins, not an infective agent, and shellfish are also invertebrates. However, as this condition is not easily classified into any other disease pigeonhole, it is generally accepted as being a zoonosis.

Other afflictions, such as malaria, which might be assumed to be zoonoses, are not considered by experts to be so, as malarial mosquitoes are only a vector for the disease, with the reservoir of infection being infected individuals within the human population. The confusion arises as some animals can be a temporary alternative food supply for the mature mosquito but do not show clinical signs of suffering from the disease in significant numbers. This is not true of some other mosquito-borne infections, such as West Nile virus, where the infective reservoir may be one of many animal species, and is therefore a true zoonosis.

Causative pathogens

The causative organisms responsible for zoonoses consist of a heterogeneous group. As can be seen from Table 1.1, they cover a very diverse collection of organisms representative of many classes of pathogens.

Table 1.1 Types of causative agent

Types of causative agent	Examples
Arthropods	Scabies (also as vectors)
Bacteria	Brucellosis, tuberculosis
Fungi	*Cryptococcus*, ringworm
Helminths	Ascariasis, *Toxocara*
Prions	BSE/vCJD
Protozoa	Toxoplasmosis, cryptosporidia
Rickettsia	Q fever
Viruses	Ebola, rabies

BSE, bovine spongiform encephalopathy; vCJD, variant Creutzfeldt–Jakob disease.

The range of symptoms and effects they produce in both their animal hosts and humans are just as diverse, ranging from the asymptomatic, through the slightly inconvenient, to mortality in excess of 50% of infected individuals. This can reach more than 90% in an outbreak of Ebola virus, which fortunately is not native to Europe, and is rare in its normal range of sub-Saharan Africa. An outbreak which began in Gulu district in northern Uganda during the autumn of 2000 had claimed 150 lives by early December, including many healthcare workers.[1]

It can be seen that the causative pathogen of a zoonosis usually comes from a class of organism capable of causing disease in single-species groups. The important difference between those pathogens responsible for zoonotic disease and other members of the same group or family of pathogens lies in their ability to cause disease across at least two species groups, of which human beings, implicitly by the definition of a zoonosis, must be one.

This is the one common factor in all pathogens responsible for zoonotic infections. Regardless of their type, they must have this ability to cross, under suitable circumstances or conditions, between an animal and a human host. Any disease that can cross the species gap is described as having a zoonotic potential. Although this is essential, the importance of the pathogen in epidemiological or healthcare terms rests on the ease with which it makes this transfer. A highly virulent pathogen which requires extreme circumstances for transfer poses little or no threat, whereas an organism capable of transferring easily from the animal source with occasional serious sequelae in infected human patients will be significant.

Foot-and-mouth disease, although of undoubted virulence in cattle, is so difficult for a human to contract, and the necessary circumstances are so extreme for transfer to occur, that the disease is almost not zoonotic, with only 40 confirmed cases being reported to the World Health Organization in the last century. On the other side of the coin, if an extensive survey of blood donations is accurate, more than 40% of the residents of the UK have at one time or another been infected with *Toxoplasma gondii*.[2]

It is essential to recognise that only some animal diseases have a zoonotic potential, but all zoonoses have an animal host. In some diseases, although classed or viewed as being zoonoses, the animal or the humans presenting with the condition are only victims of an organism present in the environment, capable of infecting a wide number of species. The reasoning behind classifying these pathogens as zoonotic lies in the animal forming an additional and perhaps more efficient transmitter of the disease to humans than solely environmental exposure would pose. The animal host can also not just act as a reservoir of infection, but is often capable of amplifying the infection by allowing the organism to multiply.

Some organisms with a zoonotic potential do not cause a recognised disease; however, the more that investigations are undertaken, and the greater our knowledge and the outfit of investigative tools become, so the more zoonoses are identified. Changes in laboratory testing protocols, farming practice or dietary intake may also allow previously unknown organisms to move into a position where they can begin to pose a threat to human health.

A current important and relevant example of a pathogen under intensive investigation would be *Mycobacterium avium* var. *paratuberculosis*, the causative organism of Johne's disease in cattle worldwide. Infection in humans with *Mycobacterium avium* var. *paratuberculosis* and development of Crohn's disease have been anecdotally linked for many years and transmission from cattle to humans by ingestion of infected dairy products has been demonstrated. Arguments between experts in the field continue over the evidence relating to the clinical role of the bacterium, with no firm conclusion as to causal linkage. The organism is difficult to culture in the laboratory as it is notoriously slow-growing and requires optimal conditions. This may partly explain why it has been isolated from only some samples obtained from Crohn's sufferers, and not all. Following the Fifth International Colloquium on Paratuberculosis in Wisconsin, USA, and the development of genetic pathogen fingerprint tests, much research is being undertaken to determine or disprove any linkage between the affliction and the organism.[3]

Linking cause and effect can be difficult because of the long incubation or prepatent period associated with some zoonotic diseases. Infection with Lyme disease, a tick-borne zoonosis of deer, may only become evident in humans when the serious sequelae of cardiac damage, neuropathies or arthritis appear many years afterwards. Many cases of zoonoses go undetected or resolve spontaneously, often due to antibiotic use for another condition, destroying the zoonotic organism before the end of the prepatent period, or before clinical manifestations appear. With blind usage of broad-spectrum antibiotics becoming less common as part of antimicrobial resistance strategies, the use of specific agents against cultures of sensitive organisms will emerge as the norm. It is possible that this will lead to more cases of long prepatent zoonotic disease and an increase in clinical significance, as there will be a failure to eradicate the pathogen before it can pose a risk to susceptible infected individuals.[4]

There is a need for the significance and scale of infection with some zoonotic pathogens to be evaluated. Until screening for *Chlamydia* and *Toxoplasma* was developed it was impossible to determine the incidence of these infections in pregnant women. Many cases of spontaneous abortion attributable to these pathogens had been blamed on a wide range of other causes. It was only with retrospective investigations of serological markers that the true incidence of infection and causal attribution could be made. These investigations have allowed the development of harm-reduction and prevention strategies which, coupled with health information campaigns, have reduced the significance of these diseases for human morbidity and mortality.[2]

Routes of transmission

A potential zoonosis may not necessarily cause detectable symptomatic disease in the animal host, nor is transmission to humans certain from every exposure to the pathogen. As with any other infection, the size of inoculum necessary to initiate progress to clinical disease varies from causative organism to causative organism, and also depends on the route of transmission. The level of inoculum necessary in an infection of a human by *Yersinia pestis* (plague, Black Death) is believed to be a single bacterium delivered by a bite from an infected flea. This is exceptional and stems from infection occurring by direct injection of the organisms into the blood stream, and also the aggressiveness of the pathogen concerned. Moderate-sized inocula or repeated infection with small cumulative amounts of pathogen are considered to be more the norm. An exceptionally large inoculum may be necessary in certain types of food poisoning. Necrotic enteritis or pigbel is caused by the ingestion of large quantities of the exotoxin from *Clostridium perfringens*, with or without the living organism being present. In most recorded cases the infective dose of the toxin is estimated to be produced by >10^8 cells of the pathogen. The ensuing intestinal damage caused by the toxin, with overwhelming colonisation of the gut either by the associated pathogen or other opportunistic bacteria, leads to septicaemia which may be rapidly overwhelming, with fatal outcome.[5]

The mode of transmission varies from zoonosis to zoonosis and can also vary for the same causative organism from host species to host species (Table 1.2). Transmission from animal to human can be not only by direct, but also by indirect contact. Indirect spread by physical contact with a previously infected object or surface is known as fomites spread.

Table 1.2 Mode of transmission

Aerosol inhalation
Blood, saliva
Faeces, urine
Fomites (contact)
Food and water
Oral or physical contact
Parasitic vectors (fleas, mosquitoes, lice, ticks)
Scratches, bites or wounds
Skin, hair or wool

Indirect spread may also involve animal-associated organic residues, such as urine, faecal matter or tears and nasal secretions. *Chlamydia psittaci* can be spread by inhalation of dried bird faeces and causes psittacosis (ornithosis) in humans – the parrot's disease of comedy. A serious clinical case is no laughing matter for a human victim, as it can lead to serious sequelae in rare cases. The same pathogen is also endemic in sheep, where it is transferred to humans by contaminated fluids or tissues.

It is also worth noting that the disease presentation and clinical course associated with this particular causative organism varies depending on the route of infection. The zoonotic pathogen that offers the most dramatic illustration of how dissimilar a disease pattern may be caused is *C. psittaci*. The form of the illness associated with infection acquired from birds usually appears as a flu-like illness with fever and chills followed by pneumonia. It rarely causes systemic disease; however, it can progress to a septic form with hepatitis, endocarditis and ultimately death. By contrast, infections of sheep origin can demonstrate rapid progression to systemic disease with serious consequences, especially in pregnant women. Colonisation of the placenta occurs and can be fatal for mother and baby, with late term abortion and neonate death. This particular pathogen is virulent enough that the most indirect contact can be sufficient to spread the disease. Following investigations of reported cases, pregnant women whose partners work in close contact with sheep are advised not even to handle unwashed overalls which may be contaminated with blood or secretions from ewes or lambs, and wherever possible to avoid contact with pre-, peri- or postpartum ewes or young lambs.

In most diseases infection is by more obvious routes. The transfer of whole blood or exuding plasma forms a very effective and direct transmission route for many pathogens. Farcy or glanders caused by *Pseudomonas mallei* is seen in humans following contamination of cuts and grazes by exudate from wounds on horses. Jockeys or stable hands in countries where the disease is endemic are especially at risk. Although the last case was seen in the UK in 1928, the disease is still seen in Europe and overseas. Horse racing and other equine pursuits are international, so there is a potential risk to the growing number of leisure horse owners and riders who may not be aware of the significance or risk that this infection may pose, and may choose to ride whilst abroad.

Ingestion of contaminated foodstuffs or water also offers an effective route for a zoonotic pathogen to cross the species barrier. Unpasteurised milk has historically been recognised as a source of several important zoonoses. Classic tuberculosis (*Mycobacterium bovis*) of animal origin was spread widely in the past by infected dairy produce. The introduction and refinement of a system of milking, storage, treatment and distribution with strict temperature and bacterial monitoring, coupled with establishment of a comprehensive herd-screening programme, has virtually eliminated the bovine-derived infection from the human population. In the 1830s, when the first Euston station was built on a site previously occupied by a particularly infected and disreputable urban dairy, several medical authorities of the day claimed the demolition of the dairy to be one of the most significant factors in an observed reduction of infections linked to the consumption of milk by young children in London. It was not until 1882 that Koch identified the causative organism in milk and that any major advances were made in prevention strategies.[6]

Tuberculosis is not the only disease that can spread by this route. Milk can also carry the causative organism of Q fever (*Coxiella burnetii*), which usually causes a mild illness similar to flu, but in rare cases can cause pneumonia, hepatic and cardiac damage, and death. The use of effective pasteurisation is still tremendously important in preventing disease spread from this source; however, on occasions system failures can allow pathogens to survive and wreak havoc.

Meat, especially poorly cooked or incorrectly stored comminuted meat products such as beefburgers or sausages, can carry a wide variety of organisms, some responsible for potentially harmful zoonotic infections. The pathogens usually cause self-limiting diarrhoea and other gastrointestinal disturbances in otherwise healthy subjects, but can be fatal for already debilitated individuals. There is believed to be dramatic underreporting of food poisoning, with an estimated 10 cases for every one of the approximately 98 500 reported to the Public Health Laboratory Service in the year 2000.[7]

At present the most significant zoonotic disease, and certainly the one most exercising the imagination of the British public and healthcare professionals, is the dietary and societal impact of bovine spongiform encephalopathy/variant Creutzfeldt–Jakob disease (BSE/vCJD) linked to the consumption of beef derived from infected cattle. The theory that this disease is caused by a prion is now fairly widely accepted as the most likely explanation for the pattern of infection and disease. A prion is defined as a polypeptide entity with no nucleic acid, consisting solely of a sequence of amino acids. Once into the body of the host it is capable of replicating intracellularly, especially in nervous tissue, and following migration, leads to the development of a spongiform encephalopathy, where the brain and central nervous system are affected. On autopsy, the appearance of areas of the brain is similar to a sponge. Proteinaceous sheets are found in the remaining cell structure and large vacuoles or spaces in between the sheets give confirmation of the diagnosis. The emergence of this disease has had a profound effect on the meat and livestock trade, from farmer to retailer. The ultimate death toll is hard to predict, and the final analysis of the current outbreak will only be possible in the future.[8]

Other organisms associated with the ingestion of infected meat and meat products have also hit the headlines. *Salmonella enteritidis* infections from a chain of Chinese takeaways in Lanarkshire was a nine-day wonder and caused several people to receive hospital treatment. However, the most significant and deadly outbreak of the last decade was the outbreak of *Escherichia coli* (enterohaemorrhagic *E. coli* or EHEC) 0157 linked to J Barr, butchers and bakers, of Wishaw,

Scotland. The total fatalities associated with the outbreak reached 21 following the consumption of contaminated meat products. This, and later outbreaks of the same pathogen in Cumbria and Scotland, coupled with a survey revealing the lack of knowledge displayed by the general public relating to the safe storage and preparation of food, led to the establishment of the Food Standards Agency (FSA). At present the FSA has taken on the role of watchdog and educator. It is responsible for making policy and enforcing standards across the food industry in production, distribution and retailing.[9]

An attempt is also underway to introduce lessons on food safety in secondary schools to address the lack of understanding and knowledge. Until the level of education of the public at large relating to the handling, storage and cooking of food improves, it is likely that further high-profile cases of infection related to food-borne zoonoses will occur.

Physical damage of the skin or body tissue can lead to open wounds capable of acting as a window for opportunistic pathogen transfer. The obvious individuals likely to fall victim to infections from this route of infection are people who handle animals in the course of their work, be they agricultural workers, veterinary surgeons or animal rescue workers. A less obvious group at risk from this mode of transmission is any pet owner, especially those foolish enough to allow their animal to kiss or lick them. Anybody who is bitten or scratched by an animal is placed at an increased risk of contracting zoonotic diseases. Rabies, fortunately currently not present in the UK but widely distributed in continental Europe, the Americas, and most of the rest of the world, can be transferred by the bite of an infected animal. Scratches inflicted by an infected cat can transfer *Bartonella henselae*, the causative organism of cat scratch disease to humans; however, there have also been reported cases where owners have been foolish enough to allow cats to lick their open wounds.[10]

Physical contact does not pose a risk just from the living animal. Animal skins, hair or wool can act as a physical reservoir, particularly in anthrax. Once known in its pulmonary form as woolsorter's disease, infection can occur following inhalation of spores from infected fleeces during processing. A recent case in August 2000 in Bradford in a textile worker is a striking example of re-emergence of a supposedly eradicated condition. Currently customs officials in the USA and the UK are impounding goatskin bags brought from Haiti by tourists as these have also been found to carry anthrax spores.

Touching an object or surface which has been in physical contact with an infected animal can also lead to infection. This is known as fomites spread and is significant in ringworm, and anthrax in its cutaneous form. The inoculum on the fomites may consist of active organism, spores or encysted forms. Following infection, surface colonisation may occur, or disease progression may occur after the introduction of the initial inoculum into wounds or inhalation or ingestion.

Contamination of water or food by faecal matter or urine causes many infections. Direct ingestion of faecal matter, especially by children, can also occur. This process, known as pica, is especially significant in infection with *Toxocara* and *Toxoplasma gondii*. Weil's disease, caused by *Leptospira* spp., follows consumption of water contaminated with either infected equine or rodent urine. Such consumption may be unwitting or accidental, and is commonest amongst devotees of water sports and other outdoor pursuits. Many cases of Q fever are related to the occupational exposure of stockpeople to the infected urine of cattle in their charge.

Transmission of zoonotic pathogens may also be caused by the involvement of vector species, particularly fleas, mosquitoes, lice or ticks. Physical contact with animals can lead to transfer of arthropod vectors; however, these vectors can also be encountered in the wider environment. Once infected, arthropods may act not only as an infective vector; they may also act as a persistent or temporary reservoir of infection with vertical transmission from generation to generation from infected mother to her eggs (transovarian transfer). Interestingly, controlling the arthropod vector is usually the mainstay of prevention in many of these infections, as without the vector, humans and infected animals may occupy the same geographical area without disease transfer taking place. The absence or control of the vector may not arrest the disease in the animal host; however, it can prevent or reduce the spread into the human population. The spread of Lyme disease from deer to humans in the UK occurs mainly through being bitten by a hard tick *Ixodes dammini*. In areas where it is endemic, clearance of low vegetation in woods and around footpaths where the tick loiters awaiting its next victim reduces infection rates.[11]

Flea control by the use of insecticides or development-arresting agents in both domestic and commercial settings is not only effective at preventing the irritation associated with the mental and physical effects of the bite, but is also important in the control of possible zoonoses. Fleas are usually host-specific, especially as adults, when the female will try to obtain a blood meal only from a preferred host; when the preferred host is not available, they will prey on any warm-blooded host. It is therefore not sufficient to control fleas but also the normally associated host must be controlled. This is particularly important in arresting the spread of *Y. pestis*, the causative organism of plague, where both rats and their fleas need controlling.

Mosquitoes can also be vectors in the spread of specific zoonoses. The recent outbreak of what was initially believed to be St Louis encephalitis in New York, USA, was later identified as West Nile virus carried by migratory birds. Transmission to humans follows the bite of infected *Culicoides* mosquitoes, which had previously obtained a blood meal from a diseased bird. An increase in the number of mosquitoes in the urban New York area had followed discontinuation of pesticide spraying on areas of standing fresh water, including Central Park, where mosquito larvae develop. Weather conditions were also believed to be partially to blame as more migratory birds, which carry the pathogen, were found in New England, having been blown off course by adverse winds, and remained resident due to continued bad weather.[12]

Humans preyed on by a vector are only infected if the vector has previously bitten an infected normal host. In most cases the vector is essential for the pathogen to cross the species barrier. Controlling the vector can therefore stop or slow transmission and spread of the pathogen, and its associated disease. Once across the species barrier infection spreads within the human population, following similar pathways to any other diseases if the pathogen has the potential for human-to-human transmission. These can include physical or sexual contact, inhalation and ingestion.

Importance of zoonoses

The importance of zoonoses in terms of human health and well-being cannot be underestimated. They affect how we live our lives, not only in a narrow health-related sense but also in a much wider cultural context. The threat that zoonotic diseases pose has shaped human history and many aspects of the infrastructure of our physical and social environment, including:

- Animal welfare – both domesticated and wild
- Food safety
- Public health and hygiene

The earliest encounters of humans and zoonosis probably occurred before the beginning of written history. Handing on to the next generation the knowledge necessary to avoid illness or death from such diseases, in association with measures necessary to control other illnesses, forms part of certain religious conventions and proscriptions. This is particularly true when we consider food-borne zoonoses. The rules relating to food preparation and consumption within halal or kosher disciplines and secular folk tradition encompass measures which can be linked to prevention or limitation of the spread of diseases, including certain zoonotic infections.

Any infection stemming from an organism occurring in a foodstuff of wholly animal origin, present in the animal or its products at the time that it is 'harvested', is considered to be a food-borne zoonosis. In the past the risks associated with consumption of food were an accepted part of day-to-day living and dying. Today, with greater life expectancy, the desire for and reality of a cleaner and safer environment, mortality associated with such diseases has become unacceptable.

In modern western society much traditional knowledge has been lost with social changes and fragmentation of family and social structures. A lack of knowledge in the majority of the population of basic food hygiene, coupled with our more extensive diet and demand for cheap food, has led to the situation where the safety and availability of our food supply are not so much dependent on the turn of the seasons, but on specialised transportation, storage and the application of modern farming methods. Supply of foodstuffs is globalised, with fresh produce being air-freighted and shipped by sea as well as by land. The supply chain has lengthened dramatically, and the need for clean 'harvesting' and appropriately monitored transportation has never been greater. Storage of produce, either as raw material or processed product, at correctly maintained temperatures has become essential in protecting the public from a whole range of pathogens, including some zoonoses.[13]

The changes in agricultural practice are particularly significant in relation to the re-emergence of certain zoonoses, as many modern animal varieties are bred to suit mass-marketing conditions and mechanisation of processing. The development of these breeds and the methods of feed and housing to optimise production often give rise to individuals with a decreased immunity, or a higher population of pathogens. The increased risk that such individuals pose to the wider animal population has been reduced by the widespread use of antibiotics as growth promoters. There are increasing concerns that the use of antibiotics in agricultural production, especially those moieties used or related to those used in human medicine, is leading to the emergence of resistant pathogens. Some of the more significant of these pathogens have a zoonotic potential, or are existing recognised causatives of zoonoses. The organism with probably the most developed resistance to antimicrobials is *Salmonella typhimurium* DT104 R serotype. This had been found to be resistant to ampicillin, chloramphenicol, streptomycin, sulphonamides, tetracyclines, trimethoprim and the quinolones. A systematic review of the use of such agents is currently being undertaken by the Department for Environment, Food, and Rural Affairs (DEFRA). This will probably cause major changes in agricultural industry practice in the UK; however, it is unlikely to affect many other countries' use of these substances in agriculture. The previously mentioned globalisation of the food market may become increasingly significant in our attempts to manage antibiotic-resistant strains of bacterial pathogens.[14]

Much of the legislation in agriculture and the food-handling industry stems from the need to deliver a safe product to the consumer. Failures in systems or inspection procedures can lead to contamination of the production and supply chain. This in turn can lead to spectacular outbreaks, sometimes associated with fatalities, which serve as timely reminders of the need for care in handling and storing food. The Wishaw outbreak in November 1996 of E. coli O157 killed 18 people and was the second most fatal incident ever recorded from this pathogen anywhere in the world. If we include the three people who died afterwards from complications caused by the infection, it becomes the most fatal. In the aftermath, the ensuing investigation into the outbreak and the subsequent report by Sir Hugh Pennington was one of the political catalysts motivating government to establish the UK FSA. The report also highlighted the ignorance in a large proportion of the public of basic hygiene precautions relating to food storage and preparation.[9, 15]

It is important to remember that in agriculture, domesticated animals are tended for gain; they can contract zoonotic disease by its transfer from wild animal populations although sometimes links are difficult to prove, as in the possible transfer of tuberculosis from badgers to cattle. Farmers will often view zoonoses in solely monetary terms, which can have beneficial and detrimental implications for any control programmes, dependent on the financial provisions of any compensation package. When contamination with a zoonotic organism downgrades a product in quality and associated value, the agricultural industry will spend much time and money in attempting to control not only the initial infection, but also the associated disease.

Present and past eradication campaigns by either compulsory slaughter or vaccination have massively reduced the incidence of brucellosis, tuberculosis, anthrax and tetanus, which were major causes of morbidity and mortality in previous decades. It is hoped that the massive slaughter of cattle carried out following the outbreak of BSE will reduce the spread of and incidence of vCJD in the human population.

In a wider context, most of the population now lives and works in urban areas, thus having no link with the countryside or its associated industries. Therefore most people's closest encounters with animals are with those species kept as companion or leisure species in the domestic setting. The idea of our pets being a potential source of disease has also gradually become more recognised. Recommendations for pet owners on handling and caring for their animals stem from the need to control potential zoonoses and reduce infection rates. The appointment and use of dog wardens in urban areas, and campaigns by the Royal Society for the Prevention of Cruelty to Animals have reduced the number of stray dogs and cats, reducing the reservoir for many diseases.

Expanding interest in exotic animals as pets has generated its own problems. Snakes and reptiles are recognised as being the biggest population reservoir for certain unusual *Salmonella* species. As a general rule, the more exotic the pet, the more likely it is to carry unusual pathogens. Although there have been no proven clinical cases arising from a zoonotic source, it is known that armadillos are the only other species except humans that can suffer from leprosy.[16]

Responsible pet owners usually safeguard their pets through veterinary surgeon-led programmes to ensure comprehensive vaccination, worming and pest control of companion animals. Public awareness of animal welfare and the related animal health issues seems to increase with every episode of the currently popular television series involving real-life 'fly-on-the-wall' animal hospital documentaries.

Geographically, in the UK we are very fortunate. Our temperate climate and physical isolation from continental Europe, coupled with the absence of large native predators and non-human primates, make many of the physical and legislative controls very effective and reduce the possibility of outbreaks of certain zoonoses. The current quarantine regulations for the movement of animals in and out of the UK safeguard us from rabies in companion and other animals. The introduction of 'pet passports' linked to an effective vaccination programme and the electronic tagging of vaccinated animals has now commenced and is proving successful for owners and their animals and in disease prevention.

Our social infrastructure offers us protection from zoonoses and other diseases in many ways we take for granted or do not recognise. The provision of high-quality, fresh, clean drinking water confers protection against disease, including some zoonoses. Current levels of public health and hygiene, with provision of safe sewage disposal and processing, reduce the risks from water-borne organisms and environmental contamination, reducing or preventing the spreading of disease. The collection and safe disposal of domestic and industrial organic wastes also offer a high degree of protection. All these measures form part of a protective umbrella which shields us from spectacular outbreaks of diseases such as cholera and typhoid – diseases which were endemic in the UK in the 19th century, and are still seen routinely in other places around the world.

Local authority responsibility for pest control forms an important part of public protection, preventing rats, mice and other alternative hosts and their associated vectors from reaching sufficient numbers to precipitate a zoonotic epidemic.

Historically this was not always the case. The Black Death and the Plague of London were two memorable examples of epidemic zoonotic infection affecting the UK. The causative organism Y. *pestis* still kills people every year in south-western USA, Africa and Asia. We associate the spread of plague with rats; however, they are not the only associated host. Chipmunks, squirrels, dogs, cats, camels and rabbits are all able to act as alternative hosts, and their associated fleas as disease vectors.[17]

The understanding of causative organisms, their detection, classification and control have only taken place in the last century and a half. The emergence of BSE, a prion disease, is an object lesson that should teach us that, although our knowledge has advanced, we still have much to learn.

It is in the nature of human affairs that the response to control the spread, or threat of spread, of disease normally follows rather than pre-empts an epidemic or well-publicised outbreak. It is important that healthcare professionals and society in general never forget that our infrastructure and legislation, although sometimes cumbersome, shield us from much morbidity and mortality associated with zoonoses and other diseases.

Risk groups

Having discussed the threat that zoonoses pose, and the potential sources of infection, let us now turn to identifying those individuals most likely to contract disease on exposure to the pathogen. Most healthy adults with a competent immune system are unlikely to acquire a zoonotic infection at every exposure to the pathogen, even if an inoculum of potentially infective magnitude is present. In infection they are also likely to display better developed resistance to a range of possible causative organisms. This does not indicate that infection does not occur in this group – only that it is less likely than in the groups shown

Table 1.3 Main risk groups for zoonotic infection

Animal handlers
Neonates and children
Elderly and infirm
Agricultural and food industry workers
Immunosuppressed or compromised individuals
Pregnant women

in Table 1.3, who are identified by the World Health Organization as primarily 'at risk'.

In general, those most at risk are those individuals who come into daily contact with animals, are less resistant to infection, or have less regard than normal for hygiene routines. Children and the elderly have traditionally been seen as more susceptible to certain of these infections. Additionally, those individuals with a suppressed or damaged immune system stemming from whatever cause, be it infectious disease, chemotherapy or organ failure, are also at an enhanced level of risk. The realisation that animal handlers and food-industry operatives have an enhanced risk of infection or transmitting these diseases has led to health and safety legislation and recommendations on working practices to reduce risk.

Pregnant women are at risk from particular zoonoses. Information regarding *Listeria, Toxocara felis*, toxoplasmosis and chlamydial infection is now widely available from maternity services and special-interest groups such as the Toxoplasmosis Trust (see p. 56). Testing is not routinely carried out; however, individuals with particular additional risk factors, such as employment in agriculture or animal welfare, cat owners or food-industry operatives, would normally be screened for any infections likely to pose a threat to mother or baby.

Since the emergence of human immunodeficiency virus/acquired immunodeficiency syndrome (HIV/AIDS) research has shown that individuals who are immunocompromised or immunosuppressed, for whatever reason, are more at risk from a range of pathogens, including some zoonoses. Patients who have had total or partial splenectomy, are on high or prolonged doses of steroids and patients undergoing chemotherapy or radiotherapy for treatment of cancer also fall within this risk group. The diagnosis and recognition of the risk that cryptosporidial diarrhoea, psittacosis, toxoplasmosis and tuberculosis (whether avine, bovine or human) poses for immunocompromised patients have led to a process of risk reduction, and an extensive programme of education for patients and healthcare professionals.[18]

Risk factors appear to be additive in terms of associated risk from zoonoses. Any individual who falls within several of the identified risk groups has an increased risk of infection. An immunosuppressed agricultural worker who keeps pet cats and eats unpasteurised dairy products whilst being licked by a pet dog would be in considerable danger.

Genetic susceptibility may also be an additional risk factor. The pattern of transmission demonstrated by the prion responsible for scrapie in sheep appears on the best available evidence to be a good model for the behaviour of BSE in cattle and vCJD in humans. It has been established that a sheep must have a certain amino acid sequence on its genes to be susceptible to acquiring a primary case of scrapie from environmental sources. The identification of clusters of cases of vCJD in Leicestershire and Doncaster may well demonstrate the similarity in genetic make-up of the victims and offer a clue to unravelling the mystery of susceptibility and risk associated with exposure to the causative agent.

Implications for industry

In the UK, a developed system of legislation and mandatory inspection safeguards us from many zoonotic infections linked to animals and processes within our system of food production. To be effective these controls have to be enforced rigorously at all levels within the chain from the animal, through processing and distribution to the arrival at the consumer. At harvesting, routine inspection of meat, livestock slaughterhouse controls and the advisory work of the Ministry of Agriculture (now DEFRA) reduce transmission rates of many potentially dangerous pathogens. Further down the process of field to food, enforced regulation of food suppliers and vendors, sell-by dates, refrigeration and education of consumers all lead to lower levels of infection and its associated illness or mortality.

Produce loss

Uncontrolled zoonotic disease can lead to produce loss caused by poor appearance or product contamination by undesirable organisms. In the event of contamination or loss of quality, there will be an associated monetary loss, with destruction or downgrading of produce. Controlling the risk of zoonoses often requires increased inputs to gain a higher quality in the finished product so as to reach the standard required by processors, suppliers and consumers. Charging a higher price for the produce can often offset these costs; however, food pricing is a sensitive issue. In the quest for food cheap enough to compete in the global market it may be very tempting for a producer to cut corners and this can lead to outbreaks of disease stemming from inadequate or inconsistent standards of treatment or implementation.

Personnel loss

When zoonoses are present, personnel within the industry can suffer from anxiety, which may be as debilitating as the possible infection. Frank illness will often lead individual workers to change career path or employment. Long-term effects due to prolonged exposure of pathogens may lead to disability and ultimately increased likelihood of mortality where appropriate measures to control spread of disease are not in place. This places additional health and safety requirements on employers to protect their workers from these risks.

The associated issues of compensation to individuals contracting zoonoses in the work place and the issues of recruitment and retention have encouraged producers and processors to put good working practices in place.

Public impact

The impact of zoonoses on the public (Table 1.4) can be profound, especially when their knowledge and understanding are mainly fuelled by adverse and dramatic media hype. Food scares are probably the most memorable of these manifestations. Eggs, beef, milk, cheese and pork have all suffered a bad press in their turn. In many of the cases reported by the media the causative agents of the outbreak were already well known, and the problem was already being addressed before the media chose to sensationalise it. In a population dominated by an appetite for sound bites, profound fear and anxiety can rapidly be generated by such reports. The only solution to the problem is education relating to the true likelihood of infection and its associated risks.

Table 1.4 Public impact of zoonoses

Food scares with boycotts and dietary change
Increased legislation and consumer/producer costs
Public and private fear and anxiety
Morbidity and mortality
Political fallout

Media misreporting of zoonoses can be dramatic and misleading. During the recent outbreak of foot-and-mouth disease in the UK, there was an isolated news report stating that during the 1968 epidemic a man had died of the disease. An extensive search of reference books, archival material and other sources revealed no confirmation that there was any evidence of foot-and-mouth being a fatal zoonotic disease. Only two confirmed cases had been recorded in humans: one in the current outbreak and one in the last. There was overwhelming evidence that, although a wide range of animals were either susceptible to the disease or capable of acting as carriers, under normal circumstances humans were not liable to contract the affliction. No trace could be found of any report either in the UK or anywhere else in the world linking human fatalities with the disease.[19]

In desperation, a phone call was made to a friend and colleague who is a consultant epidemiologist. After he had finished laughing, he told me the following story:

> During the 1967–1968 outbreak, the Army was employed to go on to some farms to kill and destroy the livestock. On one farm, night was falling as the troops carried on the work of building and lighting the funeral pyres. The farmer and his family had vacated the farmhouse and it stood empty with all the family's possessions inside. Some of the soldiers saw a man sneaking around the buildings and then break a window and enter the house. When he re-emerged clutching items he had looted from the house they were waiting for him. When called upon to stop by the now armed soldiers, the looter decided to try and run away and make his escape, so the troops shot him. He died, not of foot-and-mouth but of high-velocity lead poisoning. His death did much at the time to dissuade other opportunist criminals from looting deserted farmhouses.

The moral of this story appears to be that when reading reports of zoonoses in the media, it is essential to remember the old adage 'Don't believe everything you read in the newspapers'. It could be argued that, although not directly responsible for the fatality, the infection was, at one remove, associated with the death, if somewhat apocryphally.

Long-term effects of food zoonoses on the public are usually confined to consumer avoidance of products perceived as suspect. Food retailers usually respond to such crises by demanding or imposing higher standards on their suppliers, which in their turn force producers to increase their inputs. Lack of confidence in foodstuffs is easily lost, and takes a long time to be regained.

Morbidity and mortality arising from zoonoses are of particular public concern. The implications for the food industry of such events have been explored earlier in this chapter; however the public impact is not confined to those who work within the various stages of the food production and food-retailing chain. Individuals may become convinced that they are going to die, regardless of the true risk, from zoonotic infections; in the last few years, several individuals have committed suicide fearing they were going to die of vCJD.

The recent cases of children dying from *E. coli* infection following an educational visit to a farm or camping in farmers' fields fuels and highlights the hysteria such cases are capable of generating. Most parents would now be extremely chary of allowing their children to go on organised agricultural visits or camping holidays. Although the statistical risk of infection is low, and the risk of mortality almost negligible, one of the less attractive facets of our society is a very obvious driver of political policy in this context. There appears to be a concerted desire within certain groups for risk reduction in normal everyday affairs to the point of absurdity. The complete absence of risk is unachievable, and would require restrictions to be placed on every aspect of human endeavour. This fallacy of a completely risk-free existence is an ever-present and all-pervading urban myth, which needs to be arrested.[15]

The realisation that education in both cerebral and physical skills is the most important factor in protecting individuals and society from the risks these diseases pose needs emphasising by all involved in the day-to-day health of the nation. There is no substitute for knowledge, whose provision and application could safeguard people far more effectively than legislation, and would also ensure that future generations lead healthy, full lives.

In general, consumer pressure groups serve a useful purpose in encouraging government and others to be responsible when crises arise. In contrast, they can also increase public aversion or panic by unrestrained and ill-informed lobbying. This is especially significant where their agenda does not coincide or is diametrically opposed to any of the other parties affected by the issue. The understandable aversion response of many members of the general public to the BSE/vCJD outbreak has resulted in many people choosing to eschew meat, and become vegetarians. As a considered decision, based upon the known facts, this was a reasonable conclusion for people to reach. The less considered and sinister aspect was the declarations made by the more extreme groups and individual activists involved in the animal rights and extreme vegetarian movements, who informed the world that this was a judgement, or punishment visited upon wicked people for their consumption of meat.

The more dramatic incidents associated with zoonoses can – especially if morbidity or mortality occurs – lead to significant political repercussions not only for entire governments and their departments, but also for individual politicians. Resignations over unwise utterances are not unknown: Edwina Currie is still best remembered for the controversy surrounding *Salmonella* in eggs, and the Ministry of Agriculture has been the graveyard for many an aspiring politician. Quick-fire legislation has peppered recent parliamentary proceedings and is often a kneejerk response to zoonotic problems. As with many measures introduced rapidly, it can often be poor-quality law, being too draconian, too complex or unenforceable.

Much of the increase in regulations associated with animal husbandry has been the result of the perceived need to introduce new systems, rather than ensuring that existing schemes were made to work efficiently and comprehensively. Often the need to be seen to be doing something outweighs the more pragmatic approach, especially where this could lead to loss of votes or position.

In conclusion, this chapter has aimed to introduce zoonoses in all their aspects, and illustrate their widespread impact on our everyday lives. An attempt has been made to set the scene for the more detailed examination in the remainder of the book. The following chapters aim to examine the more significant conditions in greater detail.

Once an awareness of these diseases is gained, it is remarkable how many chance conversations with patients, relatives or friends, snippets from radio or television, or newspaper and magazine stories become associated with these conditions. This disparate group of diseases and pathogens is of major significance in our day-to-day living and its associated processes, and it is not a matter we should ever forget or ignore.

References

1. World Health Organization. *Ebola Haemorrhagic Fever*. WHO report October 2000 and update 35 December 2000. Geneva: WHO, 2000.
2. Ministry of Agriculture, Fisheries, and Food. *Zoonoses Report UK 1999*. London: MAFF, 1999.
3. Thompson D E. The role of mycobacteria in Crohn's disease. *J Med Microbiol* 1994; 41: 74–94.
4. Smith R, O'Connell S, Palmer S. Lyme disease surveillance in England and Wales 1986–1998. *Emerg Infect Dis* 2000; 6: 4.
5. *Clostridium perfringens* gastroenteritis associated with corned beef served at St Patrick's day meals – Ohio and Virginia, 1993. *MMWR* 1994; 43: 137–138, 143–144.

6.   Greener M. Tuberculosis: out of sanitoriums and into complacency. *Pharmacoecon Outcomes News* 1998; 194: 3–4.

7.   *Statutory Notifications of Infectious Diseases; Notifications of Food Poisoning.* London: Public Health Laboratory Service, 2001.

8.   Prusiner S B. Prions. *Proc Natl Acad Sci USA* 1998; 95: 13363–13383.

9.   The Pennington Group. *Report on the Circumstances Leading to the 1996 Outbreak of Infection with E. coli 0157 in Central Scotland, the Implications for Food Safety and the Lessons to be Learned.* Edinburgh: The Scottish Office, 1998.

10. Tan J S. Human zoonotic infections transmitted by dogs and cats. *Arch Intern Med* 1997; 157: 1933–1943.

11. Kemp E D. Bites and stings of the arthropod kind. *Postgrad Med* 1998; 103: 88–94.

12. Asnis D S, Conetta R, Texeira A A, *et al.* The West Nile virus outbreak of 1999 in New York: the Flushing Hospital experience. *Clin Infect Dis* 2000; 30: 413–418.

13. Altekruse S F, Cohen M L, Swerdlow D L. Emerging foodborne diseases. *Emerg Infect Dis* 1997; 3: 285–293.

14. Threlfall E J, Ward L R, Rowe B. Increasing incidence of resistance to trimethoprim and ciprofloxacin in epidemic *Salmonella typhimurium* DT104 in England and Wales. *Euro Surveillance* 1997; 2: 81–84.

15. Advisory Committee on the Microbiological Safety of Food. *Report on Verocytotoxin-Producing* Escherichia coli. London: HMSO, 1995.

16. Salmonella *Infection and Reptiles.* PHLS press release. London: Public Health Laboratory Service, 2000.

17. Goddard J. Fleas and plague. *Infect Med* 1999; 16: 21–23.

18. Angulo F J, Glaser C A, Juranek D D, *et al.* Caring for pets of immunocompromised persons *JAVMA* 1995; 205: 1711–1718.

19. *Foot and Mouth Disease: Consequences for Public Health.* Geneva: WHO (CSR), 2001.

2

Zoonoses of companion animals

With a population of dogs and cats of 14.5 million, 1.3 million pet rabbits, 1.6 million guinea-pigs and hamsters, 3.17 million birds and 26.6 million fish, the UK deserves its reputation as a nation of animal-lovers. In a recent survey undertaken by the Pet Food Manufacturers' Association (PFMA), of the 24.6 million households in the British Isles, 48.1% owned at least one pet (Table 2.1). In the USA only approximately 34% of all households had pets of any description.

Table 2.1 Companion animal populations in the UK

Animal	Number in UK households
Dogs	6.5 million in 5.1 million households[a]
Cats	8 million in 5 million households[a]
Rabbits	1.3 million[a]
Horses	900 000 across all types[b]

Sources:
[a]The Pet Food Manufacturers' Association Survey 2000, available at http://www.pfma.com
[b]British Horse Industry Confederation, available at http://www.bef.co.uk/bhic.htm

These figures, derived from the PFMA survey in 2000 (available at http://www.pfma.com), include only the accepted classes of companion animals. People also keep pets as diverse as bats, rodents, tarantulas, reptiles and sharks.

As the population of the UK has become increasingly urban, and families have become more fragmented, companion animals have gained importance. Studies show that there is a range of benefits in terms not only of health, but also in general well-being for individuals who keep pets. The bereaved, drug addicts, mentally ill and people in long-term care settings have all been shown to benefit from animal contact.

Under a scheme run by Pets as Therapy (PAT), part of the Pro Dogs Charity (PRO), there are over 10 000 dogs and their owners who visit hospitals, hospices and residential homes regularly as therapeutic support for patients. An equivalent scheme running in Scotland is called Therapet.

The benefits of pet ownership or contact do come at a price, in terms of healthcare, especially in people suffering from certain conditions. This chapter explores the more significant zoonoses associated with the main companion animal groups. Horses are also included in this chapter, as the majority of the 900 000 horses in the UK are not working animals in the accepted sense, being mostly kept for leisure purposes.

Birds

Introduction

The species of birds kept as companion animals are extremely varied. Caged birds will often be kept as pets. Budgerigars and canaries are most popular; the PFMA estimates a population of 1 million and 360 000 birds, respectively, in the UK in the year 2000. It also estimated that there were 1.81 million other birds kept as companion animals, with everything from parrots, parakeets, cockatoos or cockatiels to racing and fancy pigeons, rare poultry, hawks and owls. Most species have at least one breed society or a network of fanciers.

The main zoonotic diseases birds can harbour are normally spread by inhalation of dried faecal material, often during cleaning out of cages or housing. Most infected people show no signs of disease; however, the elderly, young and immunocompromised are particularly at risk. *Mycobacterium avium* complex (MAC), *Cryptococcus neoformans* and psittacosis are particularly important in human immunodeficiency virus/ acquired immunodeficiency syndrome (HIV/AIDS) patients, where development of any of these diseases can be rapidly fatal.

The other major zoonosis dealt with in this section is influenza. Fortunately there has not been a major outbreak of a bird-derived, seriously pathogenic strain in the UK for a considerable length of time. The slaughter of birds in Hong Kong recently was a response to the first outbreak of a new 'pathogenic' strain, and constant vigilance is necessary to prevent a recurrence of the disastrous pandemic of 1918.

These are not the only zoonoses of birds; others can be found in the section on birds in Chapter 3, and also in Chapter 7 on emerging zoonoses. However, they are possibly the most significant in everyday healthcare.

Cryptococcosis

This is an uncommon infection in immunocompromised patients, especially those with HIV/AIDS. The causative organism is *C. neoformans*, a yeast-like fungal agent that occurs worldwide. The organism is naturally found in birds, cats and dogs, cattle, sheep, horses, plants and soil. It is an uncommon pathogen and appears to have a predilection for pigeons as it is found most commonly in these birds or in their faecal matter. It has also been found in other birds, but less frequently.[1]

Disease in animals

Although it is a rare disease in cats and dogs, it can present with skin lesions, indicating the presence of systemic disease affecting the respiratory tract and central nervous system. It is seen as an opportunistic pathogen in cats that are immunosuppressed, particularly in conjunction with feline leukaemia virus (FLV). This is a disease that progresses in cats in a similar manner to HIV in humans.

Transmission

Transmission to humans is usually by inhaled dusts and aerosols; however, there is some evidence that inoculation of wounds can also initiate infection. Healthy individuals show no clinical signs of disease, although the organism can be grown from mouth swabs, skin scrapings and gut contents. Patients who are immunosuppressed because of organic disease, e.g. HIV/AIDS or leukaemia, or long-term steroid therapy are at a small risk but significant risk of catching the disease.[2]

Disease in humans

The disease usually presents as characteristic skin lesions which are papules, usually with a necrosed centre. The skin eruptions are evidence of systemic disease, usually affecting the gut, lungs and nervous system. The disease can also present or progress as a life-threatening meningitis.[3]

Treatment

In cases of acute meningitis, the treatment of choice is amphotericin intravenously, with or without flucytosine. Alternatively, fluconazole intravenously may be used. Postinfection prophylaxis with long-term fluconazole orally is necessary for prevention of relapse after treatment.

The dose of amphotericin varies depending on the licence of the preparation used. A test dose is always given to ensure that the individual is not allergic to the drug. Therapy is then commenced on a dose/weight basis and is continued until clinical symptoms and findings are satisfactory. Flucytosine is used at a dose of 200 mg/kg in four divided doses, usually for no more than 7 days. This drug may also be used at a lower dose 100–150 mg/kg daily for at least 4 months in cryptococcal meningitis.

Flucytosine and amphotericin can cause bone marrow depression; weekly blood counts are recommended. Resistance can arise, so sensitivity testing before and during treatment is required.

Prophylaxis with fluconazole at a dose of 100–200 mg/day by mouth or by intravenous infusion begins and continues after primary therapy is complete. Women are advised to use effective contraception due to the potential teratogenicity of the drug therapy.

Prevention

As the condition is rare, blanket prophylaxis to pre-empt infection is not recommended, especially as interactions with retrovirals can complicate therapy regimes. Widespread use of antifungal drugs could also lead to the development of resistant strains.

Complete protection from the organism is not possible due to the wide range of possible animal hosts and environmental sources. Immunosuppressed patients should avoid exposure to pigeons and their faeces, especially coops or roof spaces where birds roost.

Influenza
(Flu, swine and equine influenza, fowl plague)

Influenza is a familiar name to most healthcare workers and members of the general public. In recent decades it has not been associated with massive fatalities; however, the outbreak which occurred at the end of the First World War is estimated to have killed approximately 20 million people worldwide – more than the conflict itself. Subsequent pandemics in 1957 and 1968 led to many deaths. The causative agent is an orthomyxovirus which is categorised in three types A, B and C.[4]

Disease in animals

Birds, pigs, humans and horses have been identified as reservoirs for the influenza viruses, most of which are species-specific. The organisms cycle within the susceptible species, and remain within that population. Wild populations of these creatures can also maintain the virus, with wild boar carrying different viral types to the domestic swine in the same locality. Occasionally an outbreak of pure strain virus associated with another species, such as birds or pigs, has caused human disease. It is more usual that infection in another species other than the normal host follows a mutation of the causative virus. Flocks of birds and herds of pigs can be decimated by outbreaks, which are seasonal, from viral subtypes particularly pathogenic to that species.

Transmission

Viral types A and B cause the most serious clinical disease and are sub-typed according to the two main viral proteins – haemagglutinin and neuraminidase – they carry. Influenza viruses are famous for their ability to mutate. In both types an antigenic drift following minor changes in the amino acid sequencing in the haemagglutinin portion can be observed, resulting in the structure of the virus altering gradually over a series of generations. This allows the virus to continue to be infective and avoid the development of an immune response and host immunity. Type A viruses can additionally undergo dramatic sudden changes in structure called antigenic shift. The impact of this ability is the emergence of new strains overnight with an associated possible increase in virulence or pathogenicity. All the major pandemics are believed to have been caused by type A viruses capable of circulating within and between animal and human populations, and which had undergone antigenic shift (Figure 2.1).[5]

Viral subtypes are classified not only according to protein make-up but also by their place of origin and the year in which they were isolated. The 1918 virus, commonly known as Spanish flu, is believed to have arisen from an unholy union between bird and pig strains, with a few characteristics derived from human viral types completing the mix.[6] Until recently no animal reservoir of type B viruses was believed to exist; however, now this type of influenza virus has been found in harp seals.[7]

In general, pure avian or swine-derived subtypes have a low potential to cause human disease, and although most workers in these industries can be demonstrated to have the antibodies to these families of viruses, clinical disease is rare. There are notable exceptions.

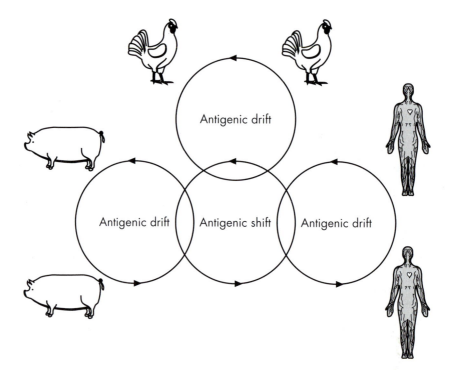

Figure 2.1 Antigenic shift and drift and the infection cycle in influenza.

In 1997 a type A virus of avian origin with a high lethality was detected in Hong Kong. A complete cull of all poultry was carried out in the region following the death of many chickens and several people. There were 20 human cases with six fatalities. The 14 survivors were seriously affected and convalescence was protracted following the infection. This was the first recorded instance of a virus of pure avian origin causing human fatalities. Another cull was carried out in 2001 after the same serotype was found to be back in circulation within the chicken population of Hong Kong. As the cull in 1997 was comprehensive, the source of the subsequent infection could either indicate another focus in a fowl population external to the area, or the maintenance of the organism in the wild bird population, as the organism has also been found in geese and pigeons.[8]

A type A virus arising from pigs caused anxiety in 1976 when it was identified in army recruits at Fort Dix in the USA. Antigenically similar to 1918 Spanish flu, fears arose that a pandemic might occur. However, the outbreak was confined to the camp and did not cause any fatalities, although it was capable of transmission from person to person and caused severe symptoms. Hong Kong was again unlucky, as in October 1999 the identification of a new pathogenic viral subtype led to a widespread cull of pigs.[9]

The World Health Organization (WHO) states that a prompt response to the emergence of new strains is essential, especially where they have high toxicity potential. The pathogenicity of any subtype stems not only from its ability to cause severe symptoms but is also related to the potential for person-to-person spread. Luckily, the Hong Kong 1997 type was shown after the outbreak to have low transmission potential, keeping the total number of cases and deaths relatively low.

Infection in animals follows the inhalation of infected aerosols. There is a fever of rapid onset, followed by cough and breathing difficulties. Copious quantities of mucus and nasal discharge are produced which, associated with the cough, produce further infected aerosols capable of continuing the infection in other individuals. Recovery is usually speedy, as is the only other possible outcome – death.

Disease in humans

In humans infection similarly follows the inhalation of infected aerosols derived from infected individuals coughing or sneezing in the immediate vicinity. There are no particular groups potentially more likely to catch the disease; the 'at-risk' groups are the very young as they have an immature immune response, the elderly, those people with asthma, diabetes, kidney or heart disease. Individuals who are immunocompromised for whatever reason are also at higher risk of complications following infection. The incubation period is usually no longer than 2–3 days. Clinical onset is characterised by fever, with temperatures as high as 40°C that may last for up to 5 days. Associated with the fever are loss of appetite, headaches, lethargy, cough, generalised joint pain, sore throat and nasal discharge. Gastrointestinal disturbance may also be seen in children. Patients are probably infective from the time that symptoms appear up to about 5 days later. As the fever starts to subside nasal congestion sets in. Convalescence normally does not extend beyond a period of 2 weeks once the major symptoms resolve; however, in the elderly and other major at-risk groups bacterial or viral pneumonia may follow, with risks of mortality. Bronchitis can also arise in individuals with previous lung damage.

Diagnosis

Diagnosis is usually symptomatic, although for monitoring purposes swabs will be cultured to ascertain prevalent subtypes.

Treatment

Treatment usually consists of simple symptomatic control. Patients are advised to rest and use suitable minor analgesics and anti-inflammatories such as aspirin, paracetamol or ibuprofen. Cough suppressants or mucolytics may also be useful. Dehydration is also a risk so patients should be encouraged to drink copious quantities of fluids.

Amantidine is licensed in the UK as an antiviral for use against type A viral subtypes as an acute treatment or as a prophylactic measure. For acute cases in children over 10 years of age a dose of 100 mg/day for 5–6 days is considered suitable. The same dose may also be used as prophylaxis in people identified as at risk but is not suitable for vaccination and healthcare workers. Prophylaxis may be extended, usually to 6 weeks or the end of an outbreak. Individuals who have been vaccinated can receive amantidine for 2–3 weeks until immunity develops. There are issues relating to the drug's use for treatment and prevention within the same household, arising from concerns over the possibility of viral subtypes developing resistance.[10]

Prevention

Due to the potential seriousness of an epidemic there is a major public health monitoring scheme for influenza in the UK. Designated general practitioner (GP) practices monitor weekly influenza and influenza-like illnesses. The Royal College of General Practitioners also collects data from GP practices. The Medical Officers of Schools Association (MOSA) monitors infection in approximately 9000 children at 35 boarding schools. The Office of National Statistics also monitors deaths from respiratory illnesses such as bronchitis, pneumonia and influenza. All of this data is coordinated by the Communicable Disease Surveillance Centre (CDSC). The Public Health Laboratory Service (PHLS) has a surveillance scheme monitoring types and subtypes currently circulating in the human population. This information, when collated for pathogenicity, case incidence and subtype, is passed to the Chief Medical Officer (CMO) and is used to drive campaigns aimed at increasing the uptake of vaccination in at-risk groups. Data are also fed into the WHO monitoring scheme.[11]

The strategy for prevention is geared to the production and comprehensive uptake of an effective vaccine. As the circulating subtypes of influenza have the potential to mutate rapidly, preparation has to be predicted on emerging and current subtypes. The WHO makes the decision in February of any year as to which subtypes should be used as the basis for the vaccine. This decision is based on the data it derives from its monitoring laboratories in London (UK), Atlanta (USA) and Melbourne (Australia). Following the decision, vaccine manufacture begins immediately, and is released in the autumn of the same year. The effectiveness of the vaccine hinges on the sophistication and accuracy of the prediction and monitoring system. Production of the vaccine starts in March each year and continues throughout the spring and summer. During the autumn of 2000 eight million doses of vaccine were produced and administered in the UK.

Those individuals considered to be suitable and most likely to benefit from vaccination are those already identified as at-risk, excluding young children and with the addition of workers in social and healthcare services. It is particularly important that the elderly in long-stay residential accommodation are vaccinated as a localised outbreak has the ability to spread rapidly. Physically fit adults under 65 years of age are not considered to need immunisation unless they are healthcare workers.

Individuals identified as at-risk should be encouraged to stay at home rather than frequent public places during epidemics to avoid infection.

A therapeutic advance in the treatment of influenza (both types A and B) has been the arrival in the market of a new antiviral agent zanamivir (Relenza: Glaxo Wellcome). A neuraminidase inhibitor, it is licensed for therapeutic use in the UK. Available as a dry powder inhaler with 5-mg blisters, the recommended adult dose is 10 mg twice a day for 5 days.

Therapy has to be initiated as soon as possible after exposure and no later than 48 hours after the onset of clinical symptoms. The data available suggest that the duration of the infection can then be reduced by a day or several days, depending on how quickly it is used. The neuraminidase, an enzyme, prevents the virus from migrating from infected cells to the rest of the respiratory tract.

It is unclear as yet what role this drug will have in overall influenza prevention strategy. Following the decision by the National Institute for Clinical Excellence (NICE) to allow it to be dispensed within the National Health Service, and its appearance in patient group directions in some health authority areas, results are awaited.

In agriculture, importing poultry from areas where avian influenza is endemic is prohibited under the Animals and Animal Products (Import and Export) (England and Wales) Regulations 2000 and the Products of Animal Origin (Import and Export) Regulations 1996. All poultry, hatching eggs and poultry meat must be declared free of avian influenza and other notifiable diseases by the producer and the importer. When the Ministry of Agriculture is informed of an outbreak, a declaration may be made by the Minister making it an offence to import specified animals and/or animal products from the affected country or region. This led to the banning of eggs and poultry from some regions of Italy during 2000. The regulations appear to work, as the last outbreak of avian influenza was recorded in the UK in 1992.[12]

The Department for Environment, Food and Rural Affairs (DEFRA; previously the Ministry of Agriculture, Fisheries, and Food) and Health and Safety Executive (HSE) advice to poultry workers is that they should wear protective clothing, including respirators, wherever and whenever fowl plague is present in flocks. This is good practice at any time.

Mycobacterium avium complex

Tuberculosis or TB is classically caused by *Mycobacterium tuberculosis*. The term is often used to describe a complex of infection states caused by a variety of aerobic bacteria of the genus *Mycobacterium*.

Several sections in this book deal with various members of this genus, some of which are associated with various diseases states which are often classified under this umbrella term. As the first section dealing with this family of microbes, there are also some general remarks relating to these infections.

General remarks

Mycobacteria are aerobic, Gram-positive bacilli found widely in a variety of animal species, including humans, and also free-living within the environment. They are intracellular-dwelling and are particularly capable of developing resistance to a variety of antimicrobial agents. The most significant members of the genera in terms of possible zoonotic infections are *M. bovis* (found in cattle, dogs and pigs), *M. avium* (found in birds, pigs and sheep) and *M. marinum* (found in seals, sea lions and fish). *M. tuberculosis* is mainly found in humans and the infection circulates within that population. For this reason it is not seen as a zoonotic disease, although it has been isolated from primates, cattle, dogs, pigs and parrots.

In general, mycobacteria are transmitted from infected individuals, be they humans or animals, primarily by the aerosol route. Infection is also possible via contact with, or ingestion of, infected tissue, bodily secretions or body fluids such as blood or plasma. Cutaneous inoculation is also possible via cuts or lacerations.

After infection there can be a short or long prepatent period depending on the health of the individual and the strain and virulence of the organism. The disease progresses, with the organism becoming disseminated throughout the body. Major sites of colonisation are usually the lungs, lymph nodes, circulatory system, liver, spleen and other major organs. Signs and symptoms vary depending on the main sites of infection. The classic tubercular lung disease usually presents as a persistent cough that does not resolve. As the condition worsens, quantities of mucus are produced which may contain traces of blood. As pulmonary damage worsens, coughing overt blood (haemoptysis) is seen. Other symptoms include loss of appetite and anorexia, fever that may be episodic, weariness and extreme fatigue. It is thought that the 'consumption' of the last centuries, immortalised in romantic fiction and drama by leaving the hero or heroine of the piece dying dramatically, was probably pulmonary tuberculosis. The disease can also manifest in a cutaneous form with ulcers and lesions progressing to persistent suppurative sores.

M. avium is endemic in wild and caged birds and, coupled with *M. intracellulare*, it can cause a form of tuberculosis with both pulmonary and systemic forms in susceptible humans. This is known as *Mycobacterium avium* complex or MAC. It is a major clinical problem in immunocompromised patients and is one of the marker infections in the progression of HIV infection to AIDS-related complex (ARC). There is some debate whether MAC is a zoonotic infection as the pathogen is widespread in the environment and some isolates display different serological profiles to classic bird-borne types. However, there is some evidence that infection may spread from birds in occupational and domestic settings.

In addition to the well-documented manifestation of MAC in HIV/AIDS, there is currently a discussion taking place as to the possible involvement of *M. avium* in Crohn's disease. Clinical links are as yet unproven.

Transmission

Transmission of *M. avium* usually occurs by inhalation of infected aerosols or dusts. Sneezing or coughing birds with subclinical cases can be prolific excreters of viable organisms. Ingestion or cutaneous contact has been postulated as an alternative route of infection; opinion is divided on the importance of this particular mode of infection.

Disease in humans

Infection usually starts with the development of foci in either the lungs or gastrointestinal tract. Disseminated infection may develop from these foci, with an associated morbidity and mortality, especially in cases of advanced HIV.

Diagnosis

Diagnosis is often presumptive as *M. avium* can cross-react to skin testing for other mycobacterial conditions. Isolation and culture are difficult due to the intracellular nature of the bacterium; however, this does produce a definitive diagnosis and also allows drug-sensitivity testing.

Treatment and drug prophylaxis

There are specific problems with antimicrobial-resistant serotypes in this infection. This is especially important in immunodeficient patients. There are also additional complications relating to dose adjustments of other concomitant drug therapies when treatment or prophylaxis for MAC is necessary. For this reason patients with MAC are not normally initiated on drug therapy in primary care. The *British National Formulary* (*BNF*)[13] recommends that expert advice is sought and patients need to be carefully assessed in secondary care settings before therapeutic decisions are made.

Strategies for treatment and prophylaxis in the UK use a new rifamycin, rifabutin. Treatment is based on a dose of 450–600 mg of rifabutin daily as a single dose for up to 6 months until sample cultures are negative for the organism. Adverse effects of the drugs used in therapy may mimic MAC infection and so the progress of treatment has to be monitored by culture and on serological findings.

By contrast, in the USA an alternative regimen is used with a macrolide antibiotic, either clarithromycin or azithromycin, being considered suitable alone or in combination with rifabutin. The premise for the use of this combination therapy is that it reduces the risk of producing drug resistance and also of secondary infections.[14]

Before prophylaxis is initiated, disseminated MAC disease should be ruled out by clinical assessment. There are concerns that treatment with rifabutin could result in the development of cross-resistance to rifampicin in persons who have active tuberculosis caused by *M. tuberculosis*. Therefore it is necessary that appropriate testing is carried out with a negative finding before rifabutin therapy is commenced.

Prophylaxis aimed at preventing the development of disseminated MAC is recommended for patients with a CD4 cell count of less than 50 cells/μl. There is some evidence that prophylaxis can be discontinued when the CD4 cell count tops 100 cells/μl. This is a decision which must be made carefully by secondary care agencies.

In the UK, rifabutin is licensed for prophylaxis at a dose of 300 mg/day in a single dose. There is a spectrum of drug interactions which may require doses of concomitantly administered moieties or rifabutin to be adjusted. Once treated successfully, at-risk patients should be considered for lifelong therapy to prevent recurrence. Again, the regimen used in the USA is different, with the use of macrolides such as clarithromycin long-term. This therapy has some risks, as treatment with clarithromycin at a dose of 1 g twice daily has been shown to lead to a higher rate of mortality in patients than with a dose of 500 mg twice a day.[15]

Rifabutin must be administered with caution with certain protease inhibitors or non-nucleoside reverse transcriptase inhibitors used in HIV therapies. Changing agents or modifying doses is needed on a drug-by-drug basis, using latest recommendations available to optimise treatment and not compromise overall therapy. The most recent *BNF* should be used for the latest details.

Psittacosis
(Ornithosis)

Psittacosis is the classic 'parrot's disease' of comedy, although clinical cases will not have patients splitting their sides with laughter. The disease is also referred to as avian chlamydiosis (AC). The causative agent is *Chlamydia psittaci* which typically, like all other *Chlamydia* spp., is an intracellular parasite. It has a biphasic reproductive cycle, with only one phase being infectious. The same organism is also important in a zoonotic infection of sheep, although the pattern of disease and the transmission pathway are very different (see pp. 102).

Disease in animals

C. *psittaci* is widespread in both wild and domestic birds. Parrots are the most frequently encountered hosts in a companion animal setting and 1% are estimated to have active disease at any time. Other potential hosts as zoonotic reservoirs include turkeys, ducks, geese, pigeons, starlings, pheasants and birds kept for competitive showing. Estimates have been made of the prevalence of infection in wild pigeon populations in the USA. These range from half to all of feral pigeons within a population sample. The number of birds infected within a population increases where overcrowding or stress occurs. The associated levels of inadequate ventilation and cleanliness in poor and overcrowded commercial housing also promote the rate of infection with the disease in commercial flocks.

Infection in birds is usually subclinical and may remain latent for a period of months or years. Apparently healthy birds can shed viable organisms and cause infection in others during the latent period. The pathogen can survive in the environment for extended periods following contamination with infected droppings or aerosols originating from the nasal discharge of infected birds. The organism is resistant to drying, and can be found in dust in hen houses, pigeon lofts and other roosting sites. Bird cages, pet shops, lofts or roof spaces inhabited by wild and feral species must be treated as possibly contaminated.

Transmission

Transmission to humans follows inhalation of dried bird faeces or nasal discharge from infected birds, direct contact with birds or their feathers and by bird bite (a rare but possible occurrence, especially in aggressive non-domesticated parrots).[16] Once across the species barrier, human-to-human transmission may occur by the aerosol route. Poultry workers in the turkey industry, either in rearing or processing birds, show an increased incidence of the disease. Individuals who handle wild, pet or domesticated birds in any setting are at increased risk. However, obvious risk is not reliable as a diagnostic yardstick, as 20% of cases reviewed in the USA could remember no overt contact with birds. Verification of the presence of C. *psittaci* may be difficult, as the usual test does not differentiate serologically between this and other *Chlamydia* spp.

Disease in humans

The infection may be subclinical, leading to underdiagnosis. Onset of the disease is gradual; an incubation period of 1–2 weeks is followed by a series of symptoms similar to influenza or a respiratory infection. Symptoms include malaise, fever, chills and headache, and associated photophobia and a non-productive cough. An unusual feature is that, although the temperature is elevated, the pulse rate does not undergo an associated rise. Joint and muscle pain with weight loss and loss of appetite may also be seen. Occasionally a full-blown acute pneumonia may occur.[17]

Rarely seen in children, the infection is most severe in the elderly and the immunocompromised. In severe cases, liver and splenic enlargement with gastrointestinal symptoms including vomiting, diarrhoea or constipation may occur. Cardiac involvement with valve failure and endocarditis is possible. Spread into the central nervous system may follow with disorientation, depression or delirium followed by meningitis or encephalitis. Severe breathing difficulties can follow exacerbation of pulmonary symptoms. Death can follow pulmonary insufficiency and toxaemia. In clinical cases fatality occurs in approximately 1%.

Treatment

Treatment consists of tetracyclines as the antibiotic of choice, with supportive measures. Tetracycline is given at a dose of 250–500 mg three to four times daily for at least 7 days with the treatment period extended as needed. Doxycycline has also been used at a dose of 200 mg/day, as has azithromycin or erythromycin, although their use is normally associated with other species of *Chlamydia* which cause urinogenital infection or endocarditis. Early diagnosis is very important to reduce complications, and prolonged treatment may be required to prevent reinfection or relapse in some cases. The notifiable diseases section of Chapter 5 of the *BNF*[13] suggests it is good practice to inform a consultant in communicable diseases of cases of psittacosis where there could be a public health risk.

Prevention

Prevention depends on education of individuals in high-risk groups. Early detection of cases in birds is an important part of any prevention strategy. Reducing stress and overcrowding is recommended to control infective spread. Placing birds suspected of having psittacosis in isolation until they can be tested and subsequently treated or slaughtered in confirmed cases, is recommended as good working practice. Treatment of imported companion birds with prophylactic antibiotics is important, especially before their sale as pets. Good flock management at agricultural sites can reduce infection, and feral birds should be excluded from feed mills and rearing sheds. No vaccines are available for either humans or birds. There has been much discussion recently over the addition of antimicrobial substances to animal feed. In particular, the administration of some antibiotics as feed additives may control *C. psittaci* in flocks of birds. Some experts claim that barring such substances from use could lead to an increased risk of infection in the future.

Cats

Introduction

The population of cats in the UK in 2001 is estimated to have reached 8 million. This figure shows a marked increase in the number over the previous decade, and has now outstripped the dog population. This change is associated with changes in lifestyle: urban living, employment patterns and the number of single-person households have all altered the balance of ownership towards animals that require less intensive care. The PFMA (http://www.pfma.com) has estimated that 34% of households in the UK own at least one cat, with the greatest density in the south-east of England. A similar pattern is seen in the populations associated with Europe and the USA, with 47 and 75 million cats, respectively.

The reasons most frequently given for cat ownership are companionship and love, with many cat owners allowing their pets the run of their houses. Cats are capable of carrying a wide range of zoonoses and as the pattern of behaviour of certain owners falls outside the normal realms of good hygienic practice, there are many opportunities for the transfer of infection to occur.

Cats are especially significant in two well-recognised conditions, toxocariasis and toxoplasmosis, both of which pose a well-publicised risk to children and pregnant women. Cat scratch disease is now recognised as a serious condition in the immunocompromised, and the effective treatment or prophylactic therapy of cat owners with HIV/AIDS has begun to reflect the importance of this and other potentially serious zoonotic conditions.

Cats are the companion animal of choice for large numbers of the population, and therefore the control and prevention of their zoonoses are particularly important.

Cat scratch disease (CSD)

Cat scratch disease is caused by a rickettsia, *Bartonella henselae* (formerly known as *Rochalimaea henselae*). Little recognised in the UK, it is widely documented in the USA and shows a worldwide distribution. Other *Bartonella* spp. cause a number of diseases in humans, including trench fever (*B. quintana*) which occurs worldwide. *B. quintana* is transmitted to humans via bites from lice or fleas associated with rats.

Transmission

Although cat scratch disease was recognised previously as a distinct infection and illness, it was not until 1992 that the causative organism was identified because of difficulties in culturing the slow-growing bacterium. Infected cats carry the pathogen and show no ill effects; however, they can shed viable organisms, especially in their urine, for prolonged periods. In-species transmission between cats occurs by flea transmission and subsequent bites. Physical damage sustained in fighting, i.e. bites and scratches, is also believed to be a significant cat-to-cat transfer route. Recent research has indicated that a flea that sucks blood from an infected cat becomes infected. *B. henselae* replicates and colonises the flea's digestive tract; subsequently viable organisms are passed in the faeces. Cats may be infected by bacteria in flea faeces introduced into a flea bite wound or other cuts and abrasions either by scratching or grooming. This mode of transmission, of the introduction of contaminated arthropod faeces into wounds, occurs in other *Bartonella* spp. diseases and is especially important in the rodent reservoir for trench fever.[18]

Human infection follows either a cat scratch or bite from an infected animal. Saliva contaminated with flea faeces from the cat grooming itself or nibbling at the site of flea bites is presumed to be the source of the infective inoculum. The role of fleas in the direct transmission of *B. henselae* from cats to humans is unknown. Humans may also be able to contract the infection in a similar manner to cats by introducing flea faeces into either a flea bite or other wound; this hypothesis is currently under investigation.

Disease in humans

A primary lesion appears at the injury site, usually forming a single circular pink flat lesion or plaque or series of plaques along the length of the scratch. The initial primary lesion appears in 50% of cases after

10 days. Transient lymph node tenderness and swelling with some discomfort may develop and then regress. In about 15% of cases progression to more serious disease occurs with serious sequelae, which may include central nervous system damage, osteomyelitis and involvement of the lungs and respiratory tract. Immunocompromised patients may develop liver damage and hepatic lesions.[19]

Bacillary angiomatosis is a vascular proliferative form of disease seen in individuals with established HIV or who are immunocompromised for a variety of reasons. It can be fatal, progressing from skin lesions, which are the most common symptom, to lesions in the bones and bone marrow, gastrointestinal and respiratory tract, lymph nodes and central nervous system. Fever, weight loss and associated swelling and tenderness of various internal organs are commonly seen. It is also suspected of causing bacillary peliosis, a condition associated with relapsing bacteraemia and endocarditis. Cystic, blood-filled spaces develop in the liver, spleen or lymph nodes. Fever, abdominal pain and weight loss follow gastrointestinal disturbance. A febrile bactaeraemic syndrome associated with *B. henselae* is also seen in immunocompromised patients. Symptoms include chronic or cyclical fever, joint and muscle pain and severe headache. Patients with long-term asymptomatic infections may shed viable organisms in their urine.[20]

Treatment

Treatment in simple cases is usually using rifampicin, ciprofloxacin or trimethoprim at maximum dosage levels. In cases with complications, erythromycin or doxycycline for long-term therapy may be required to prevent relapse and effect a full cure. Controlling cat fleas may well prevent cats contracting the disease and reduces the chance of transmission to humans. A regular programme of insecticide use with other measures should be considered.

Prevention

Owners are advised to avoid rough play with cats to reduce the risks of scratches and bites. Any wounds inflicted by the cat should be washed and disinfected immediately. The common-sense precautions of preventing a cat licking any human wound and washing any exposed areas after petting or stroking the cat are strongly recommended. Children and adults, especially those who are immunosuppressed, should avoid stroking or touching stray or feral cats. Immunocompromised patients, especially those with advanced HIV or with ARC, may need to consider keeping their cat indoors at all times to prevent it associating with other cats which may be infected.

Hookworm
(Ancylostomiasis; cutaneous larva migrans; creeping eruption)

The hookworms *Ancylostoma duodenale, A. braziliense, A. caninum* and *Necator americanus* are associated with two clinical conditions affecting human beings. The adult worms are found in the gut of cats and dogs and the eggs are passed in the faeces to the soil. Under suitable soil conditions the eggs remain viable for considerable periods. Once hatched the eggs produce larvae which undergo two larval moults in the soil. On attaining the third larval stage they become infective. They can penetrate intact human skin, usually at the base of a hair follicle, or are ingested by consumption of contaminated food or water. The larvae then subsequently begin to migrate. The type of migration following infection is determined by the species involved and is classified by the clinical signs seen.

Ancylostomiasis

The third-stage larval stage of *A. duodenale* or *N. americanus*, two internal parasites of dogs, is responsible for this infection. It is more common in warmer climates. Infection may be seen on exposure to infected material in the UK, but it is more commonly a zoonosis of travellers.[21]

Following penetration of the skin or if the inoculum is ingested into the gastric mucosa, the larvae begin to migrate by deep tissue penetration, and by transit via blood vessels to the lungs. They then penetrate the alveolal sacs and migrate via the bronchi and trachea, where they are swallowed into the gut lumen.

The hookworm is named for the shape and structure of its mouth parts, which aid its attachment to the blood vessels in the gut of the host, from which they feed copiously. Once in the gut they grow to between 5 and 100 mm in length and in heavy infestations can cause anaemia. The worms produce and secrete hyaluronidase so that at their site of attachment they can continue to feed freely. Even after they lose their hold or are killed by use of an anthelmintic, continued blood loss can occur due to the presence of residual hyaluronidase and its anti-coagulant effect. The worm matures in the gut and then produces eggs which are passed in the stools. It is unclear if some species can or cannot complete their life cycle in humans, or if they can only reach maturity in other species.

Disease in humans Symptoms of infection in humans can include pneumonia related to damage caused by the migrating worms, anaemia, nausea, vomiting, abdominal pain, bloody diarrhoea or blood in the stools and generalised weakness. Some larvae may penetrate other organs or structures than the lungs. Larvae have been found in the cornea, liver and spleen. In dogs maternal transfer to puppies is seen via the milk or through the placenta; this has never been documented in humans.

Treatment As the anaemia produced by a hookworm infection is probably the most serious effect in humans there may be a requirement for iron therapy at the same time as anthelmintic treatment. The *BNF*[13] recommends the use of mebendazole at a dose of 100 mg twice daily for 3 days. In refractive cases, where a large population of worms across larval and adult stages is present, a repeat regimen may be needed to resolve the infestation.

Cutaneous larva migrans or creeping eruption

This condition is caused by the cat or dog hookworm *A. braziliense* and also, more rarely, by *A. caninum*. It is normally seen in tropical and subtropical areas; because of the nature of the infection and its aetiology it is often seen in travellers returning from beach holidays. Many of the public beaches in the West Indies, India and Sri Lanka are known to be sources of this infection. The presentation is very distinctive and diagnosis is based on the very unusual appearance of the lesions.[22]

Disease in humans The condition is most often seen in children, as their skins are softer, especially on their feet. Clinical signs commence after penetration of the skin by the infective third-stage larvae, usually as a result of walking on contaminated sand or soil in bare feet. At the site of entry itchy reddened spots appear. After 2–3 days the larvae then commence to migrate through the germinative layer of the skin, leaving a raised red and itchy track with localised swelling (Plate 1). The track extends by several millimetres daily. Although distressing, the condition is usually self-limiting as the larvae soon die. Although only one track is usually seen, multiple tracks are also possible. In the case of multiple tracks, or where the lesion continues to advance, and in cases where a secondary infection results from scratching, therapeutic interventions may be necessary.

Treatment   The *BNF*[13] recommends that topical tiabendazole can be used to treat single tracks, although sadly no commercial preparation is available in the UK. There have been isolated reports of cattle or sheep drench wormers containing the active ingredient being obtained and used successfully, although this practice cannot be encouraged as it lies outside licensed uses. Multiple infections require the use of ivermectin or albendazole or tiabendazole by mouth, all of which are available on a named-patient basis from IDIS Ltd.

Use of any of the broad-spectrum antihistamines by mouth or as a local application will help control itching. The choice of antibiotic in secondary infection follows the usual protocol for cutaneous or sub-cutaneous infection. Flucloxacillin has been used successfully with its ability to produce adequate therapeutic levels in deep tissue. Topical antibiotics such as fusidic acid have also been used.

Prevention strategies for both conditions

As physical contact with contaminated material is necessary for infection, wearing shoes on ground which could be contaminated with dog or cat faeces is recommended. If dogs are kept in closed areas the run should be disinfected with a chlorinated or phenolic disinfectant to ensure full decontamination and destruction of any egg cysts. In the UK the passing of bylaws and associated fines encourages dog owners to clean up after their pets when they foul in public places, thus reducing contamination of the environment. The exclusion of dogs from recreation areas frequented by children and the use of dog wardens to impound stray and feral dogs is a useful measure to prevent this and other zoonoses arising from canine sources. Education of children in basic hygiene procedures helps prevent infection after exposure to the causative organism. In a holiday environment, wearing beach shoes and using beaches where dogs are excluded and sand is regularly raked and cleaned reduce the chance of exposure. Dogs and cats should be regularly wormed to eliminate the adult parasite. The emphasis is on a programme of treatment, as one animal will often have not only adult worms present in the gut but migrating larval stages at one and the same time.

Ringworm

Ringworm is a common dermatological affliction of cats, dogs, cattle and horses caused by *Trichophyton* spp. and *Microsporum* spp. of fungi. The causative organisms of ringworm are so widespread in the environment, it is often impossible to determine the source of infection. Ringworm is also known as zoonotic dermatophytosis (or dermatomycosis). The lesions are commonly circular in form and historically were believed to be caused by a worm, hence its common name. Defining the causative organism is very difficult even for expert mycologists, as there are at least four fungal species capable of affecting dogs that may cause clinical disease in canines and humans. Other carrier animals also have as many or more species of causative organism, which may be host-specific or shared between many species of mammalian host.[23]

The most common identified zoonotic organisms causing ringworm in humans are *Microsporum canis,* carried by dogs and cats, and *Trichophyton verrucosum*, carried by cattle. It is possible for pet animals to contract the disease from humans.

The picture of ringworm infection in humans is further complicated by a spectrum of organisms belonging to the genus *Tinea*. These are sufficiently ubiquitous for them to be classed as environmental pathogens. Differential diagnosis is often unnecessary before treatment begins, therefore it is sometimes difficult to determine whether infections are zoonotic or not.

Transmission

Fungal spores are shed by the animal host and are then passed to humans either by direct contact with an infected animal or by indirect contact with animal housing, fences and other contaminated fomites. Spores can remain viable for long periods of time. After infection the spores have an incubation period of approximately 10–12 days. After this time lesions may appear (Plate 2), with isolated plaques gradually forming the characteristic wheals as the infection establishes. The circular appearance is caused by the healing of the central area, whilst the organism proliferates outward. The fungus establishes in the hair follicles and may cause the hair shaft to fracture at skin level. This leads to hair loss, which may be permanent in some cases.

Established infections gradually lose the circular appearance as they progress away from the initial site of infection. The lesions are red, scaly and itchy and inflamed, oozing and crusted, especially where secondary infection following scratching occurs. Autoinfection may also result from spores trapped beneath the fingernails. Ringworm can be serious in the very young, who are specifically at risk of scalp infection which can lead to extensive rapid hair loss.

Elderly patients and the immunocompromised are also at risk: dermatomycosis causes further complications in individuals who are already suffering from a spectrum of infections and afflictions.[24]

Incidence

M. *canis* can be carried by up to 89% of asymptomatic cats. Up to 50% of people exposed to infected cats, both symptomatic and asymptomatic, have serological markers for past or present infection. Infection is more likely from animals displaying overt signs of infection.

Diagnosis

Diagnosis in animals and humans may be assisted by the use of an ultraviolet light, as the lesions will often fluoresce. Definitive diagnosis requires culture of the organism; however, this is normally unnecessary, or is not undertaken.

Treatment

The condition is usually self-limiting, but use of topical and systemic antifungals may be required. Potassium permanganate solution 1 in 10 000 is still used with considerable success, and may be considered where temporary skin discoloration is not an issue. Topical imidazole antifungal agents such as miconazole and clotrimazole are probably the most frequently used topical creams in mild cases. Terbinafine cream is usually reserved for more serious or resistant fungal manifestations. Ketoconazole shampoo may be used in scalp infections.

In persistent systemic infections griseofulvin, terbinafine or fluconazole may be necessary. Therapy usually needs to be prolonged so that the therapeutic agent can penetrate to the dermis surface in the skin cells.

Griseofulvin has passed out of use in all but the most resistant disease, as newer agents have become available. Terbinafine at a dose of 250 mg/day in a single dose offers the advantage of good patient compliance and therapy lasts from 2–6 weeks, the length of course being linked to response.

Triazole antifungals are effective oral agents. Ketoconazole by mouth has become obsolete; the Committee on the Safety of Medicines has recommended that other agents be used as there is a significant risk of liver toxicity, especially where prolonged treatment is required. Fluconazole is considered to be less toxic and is frequently used. Adult doses vary depending on severity of symptoms; for most cutaneous infections, a dose of 50 mg/day for 2–4 weeks, extended to a maximum of 6 weeks, usually effects a cure.

Therapy in immunocompromised patients is further complicated by significant drug interactions between imidazole and triazole agents and a spectrum of drugs including antiretrovirals, rifamycins, tacrolimus and certain cytotoxics. Expert advice and monitoring are essential with dose adjustments.

Prevention

Infected animals should be treated when clinical signs develop, and prophylactically where deemed necessary. Individuals identified as being particularly at risk should be encouraged to handle animals as little as possible, particularly where animals are wild or feral in habit.

Scabies

Scabies is caused by a burrowing arachnid mite, *Sarcoptes scabiei*. Recent work has demonstrated that each mammalian species has a specific race of the parasite. Zoonotic infection by mites other than of the human-specific race can be extremely irritant; however the organism does not demonstrate the ability to complete its life cycle on a human host.[25]

Disease in animals

Sources of zoonotic scabies include dogs, foxes, cats, horses and, on occasion, pigs. Infection results from close direct physical contact and also fomites spread. After zoonotic infection the mite does not burrow under the skin surface and is believed to cause itching and an associated rash solely by causing a contact dermatitis.

Feline scabies caused by *Notedres cati*, also known as notoedric mange, causes intense itching on the face, ears and neck of the cat.

Disease in humans

Feline scabies is transmissible to humans. It presents with blisters, red papules and crusting. It appears rapidly, is intensely itchy and when the lesions have been scratched crusting may be seen. Lesions appear on the areas of body in contact with the cat and are especially common on the arms, chest, legs and abdomen. Canine scabies shows a similar pattern in human infection.

Diagnosis

Diagnosis may be difficult, as in zoonotically acquired disease the distinctive burrows are absent. The usual techniques of the burrow ink test or skin-scraping examination will therefore not produce definitive results. The condition is usually of short duration, and it may be necessary to treat blindly and symptomatically. A more serious problem may be the secondary infection of the lesions by other opportunistic infections, especially in immunocompromised patients.

Treatment

Treatment using insecticides is the usual choice. Either malathion or permethrin topically applied, with the usual precautions relating to hypersensitivity, is routinely used. In cases where crusting or hyperkeratotic lesions are present repeat applications may be required. The itching is usually treated with crotamiton or antihistamine preparations. Steroids are only used to deal with any persistent dermatological reaction after eradication of the parasite.

Toxocariasis
(Visceral larva migrans and optical larva migrans)

Disease in animals

Toxocara canis and *T. cati* are roundworms of the dog and cat respectively and are found in animals worldwide. The main zoonotic reservoir is latent infections in female dogs and cats that are reactivated during pregnancy.

Transmission

T. canis is mainly transmitted from dog to dog and from dog to human by the ingestion of material infected with encysted eggs. Indirect transmission via an intermediate host is also possible. Unusually in dogs, transmission from bitch to puppies is possible via the placenta and milk. The life cycle of *T. cati* is similar, although transmission across the placenta has not been demonstrated and is believed not to occur.[26]

Toxocara demonstrates both direct and indirect life cycles in dogs, whereas in cats only the indirect cycle is seen. In the direct cycle the eggs are passed with the dog's faeces; these eggs have a variable latent period before they become infective. Eggs of *Toxocara* are extremely resistant to damage and desiccation and can remain viable and infectious in the soil for many years. The eggs may also develop into infective larvae under suitable conditions. Eggs are spherical and 75–90 μm in size.

Once mature eggs or young larvae are ingested on faecally contaminated matter, they hatch or mature through the first larval stage in the small intestine. The second larval stage (L2) penetrates the wall of the intestine into the lymphatic system and thence into the blood stream. Migration continues through the heart and lungs. In the lungs the larvae moult to the third larval stage (L3). The L3 migrate up the trachea and are ingested for a second time. Returning to the small intestine, the final moult occurs and the adult worms mate and produce eggs and the cycle begins again.

In contrast, in the indirect life cycle there is a requirement for an intermediate host, which is normally small rodents in the case of *Toxocara*. These ingest viable oocysts that subsequently hatch in the small intestine. Once the larvae reach the second larval stage (L2) they migrate and penetrate muscle tissue. A dog or cat that subsequently eats the infected rodent will become infected with the encysted larvae. Once into the gut the larvae will then migrate into the tissues of the dog or cat. They soon go back to a state of dormancy. In a bitch or queen, the dormant larvae become active during late pregnancy. Subsequently some larvae migrate to the small intestine and others migrate to the unborn pups in dogs. The cycle then starts over again, in either direct or indirect modes in the dog and in indirect mode in cats (Figure 2.2).

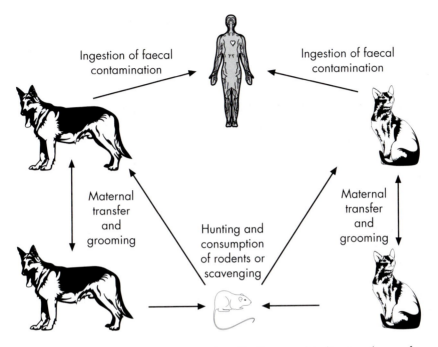

Figure 2.2 *Toxocara* transmission cycle with direct and indirect pathways from animal to animal and animal to human.

There has been some evidence in cats that reinfection may result from the cats grooming either themselves or kittens.

Disease in humans

Infection is acquired by ingesting encysted eggs (oocysts) in soil contaminated with cat or dog faeces. The eggs hatch, and larvae penetrate the intestinal wall and migrate through body tissues. In most cases, *Toxocara* infections are not serious and many people, especially adults infected by a small number of larvae, may not notice any symptoms. Annually approximately 20 cases a year in the UK are reported to the PHLS. Due to the nature of the disease and the lack of clinical signs, this figure does not represent a true picture of the number of persons infected at any time. The most severe cases are rare, but are more likely to occur in young children who often play in dirt or eat soil. Humans are a dead-end host for *Toxocara* in that the larvae that hatch from any ingested eggs cannot progress to full maturity.[27]

There are two conditions that are recognised as affecting human hosts: visceral larva migrans and ocular larva migrans.

Visceral larva migrans   Visceral larva migrans occurs when hatched larvae migrate through the body of the affected individual. The larvae may continue to migrate for up to 6 months. They finally lodge in various organs, particularly the lungs and liver and less often the brain, eyes and other tissues, where they produce eosinophilic granulomas up to 1 cm in diameter. Migration can result in multiple abscesses, hepatomegaly and pneumonitis. Symptoms include coughing, nausea, vomiting and fever, wheezing, splenomegaly and lymphadenopathy. The acute phase may last 2–3 weeks, but resolution of all physical and laboratory findings may take up to 18 months.

Ocular larva migrans   Ocular larva migrans is a rare form of visceral larva migrans that can cause blindness. The migrating larva enters the eye, encapsulates and causes a localised inflammatory reaction with the production of scar tissue (granuloma) on the retina, which may be confused with retinoblastoma. In some cases the larva can re-emerge and move within the eye structure later in life. Sufferers can experience permanent partial loss of vision. Variable degrees of ocular inflammation occur, and more severe manifestations of ocular larva migrans may require aggressive therapy to avoid serious sequelae such as glaucoma and blindness.

Treatment

Treatment relies on anthelmintic therapy with tiabendazole, mebendazole and ivermectin at normal clinical doses for both adults and children. Corticosteroids, antibiotics, antihistamines and analgesics can be used concomitantly for symptomatic relief. The ocular form may require vitrectomy with adjunctive laser treatment.

Prevention

Prevention of larva migrans in humans involves a combination of human hygiene and vigilance, stray dog and cat control (where possible), and parasite control in pets. The following hygiene measures should be adopted:

- Children and adults should always wash hands well with soap and water after playing with pets and after outdoor activities, especially before eating.
- Children should be taught not to eat soil or sand.
- Regular periodic worming treatment of puppies, kittens and nursing dogs and cats will prevent acquisition and shedding of the parasite.

- Play areas and sandpits used by children should be protected to reduce contamination from animal faeces.
- Areas which are believed to be contaminated with eggs may be disinfected using ultraviolet light or by scorching.

Toxoplasmosis

Toxoplasmosis is caused by an intracellular protozoan parasite, *Toxoplasma gondii*, which can infect any mammal and is found worldwide. It poses a well-publicised threat to human health, especially to pregnant women, and is also a significant pathogen in immunocompromised individuals. The causative organism is transmitted by contact with and ingestion of material contaminated with cysts or oocysts, especially food or water (Figure 2.3). The disease is notifiable in Scotland, but not in the rest of the UK. In 1998 there were 222 cases reported to the PHLS in England and 12 in Scotland. This is believed to represent a significant underreporting of cases.

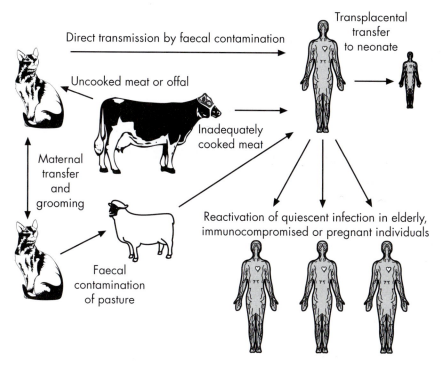

Figure 2.3 Toxoplasmosis transmission pathways.

Disease in animals

The major source of infection is cat faeces or food and water contaminated with faecal matter. The definitive hosts for *T. gondii* in which it can complete its life cycle and produce sexual oocysts are cats, either wild or domesticated. Feral cats are recognised as a significant reservoir as they hunt and consume rodents carrying the disease. Cats pass oocysts in the faeces; these become infective after a period of 24 hours, and can remain infective under suitable environmental conditions for more than a year. Sheep and goats are the main non-feline reservoir, especially pregnant or perinatal ewes, and unpasteurised milk or cheese. Infection in sheep arises from grazing on pasture contaminated with cat faeces. Any other animal then infected acts as an intermediate host.

Transmission

In an intermediate host the organism will hatch from ingested oocysts, and the invasive form or tachyzoite will actively spread into cell structures, where it proliferates and then invades the body via the blood supply. Cysts are then formed in tissues and organs, especially muscle, heart and brain. The cysts are filled with bradyzoites, a slowly maturing form, which if subsequently ingested by another susceptible animal can progress to disease. Dogs, cattle, pigs and rodents have been demonstrated to suffer from the condition and act as a reservoir. Meat from an infected animal may contain viable cysts, and thorough cooking is necessary to kill them before consumption to prevent infection. Infection by fomites transfer has been demonstrated and pregnant women should not handle overalls of people involved in lambing, nor should they handle perinatal ewes or neonate lambs. A live vaccine is available for sheep, and pregnant women are advised to avoid handling the vaccine or any recently vaccinated sheep. Contaminated material containing viable oocysts introduced into open cuts or wounds can also act as an inoculum.

Disease in humans

Although infection is common in humans – some surveys report that more than 50% of adults show immunological markers – the associated disease is fortunately less common, and does not pose a risk except in particular circumstances. Children or adults infected for the first time may well present with a generalised lymphadenopathy which is self-limiting and resolves after a few weeks, leaving the individual resistant to infection, with possibly low numbers of encysted organism in tissue or organs and persistent serological markers. Once infected, an individual can carry the cysts asymptomatically until reactivation occurs, especially in immunosuppressed patients. As with animals, the cysts are usually located in skeletal muscle, heart or brain tissue.[28,29]

Pregnant women who contract toxoplasmosis shortly before or after conception are at a much higher risk and need to be treated to prevent transplacental spread to their unborn child, which can occur in 40% of clinical cases. If the infection passes to a neonate or unborn child a congenital infection can follow with profound effects from systemic disease. Dependent on the point that infection occurred there may be severe neuropathological changes. Infection in early pregnancy can lead to miscarriage, stillbirth or a neonate with hydrocephalus or retinochondritis, which is an inflammatory condition of the retina and chondron in the eye. Nystagmus or squint may also be present, as may also be brain calcifications that can precipitate seizures and epilepsy. Later infections are unlikely to lead to miscarriage but may lead to premature delivery. Damage of similar types to early infection may be present or develop postnatally.

Pregnant women in the UK are not routinely tested for toxoplasmosis. Testing is encouraged if they belong to a high-risk group such as cat rescue workers, those employed in agriculture or those who have cats as pets. A concerned pregnant woman can also request a test, although the risks and limitations of the test should be explained. Testing can demonstrate whether infection is recent or historical. In a mother with an active infection amniocentesis or chorionic villus sampling or biopsy can determine whether the fetus is infected, and ultrasound scans may determine the extent of any damage. Both amniocentesis and chorionic villus sampling carry a 1% risk of the testing procedure causing spontaneous abortion; however, there is a major difference between the techniques when termination may become necessary. Chorionic villus sampling is not carried out before 12 weeks after conception because there have been incidents of fetal abnormality arising from the technique: results can be determined 2–3 days after sampling, allowing suction termination where required. This is not the case with amniocentesis, where the technique cannot be carried out before 16 weeks, and results take 2–3 weeks to obtain. This can lead to the need for very late term termination, with the associated problems and issues that this raises.

In the event of damage being confirmed, a termination may be offered. A baby born to a perinatally infected mother will require postnatal follow-up. It is worth noting that the Medical Defence Union has stated that refusal to test a pregnant woman who has requested such a test and who subsequently produces a congenitally infected child is potential grounds for a negligence claim.

Toxoplasmosis can also cause a poorly recognised prolonged illness with acute episodes, which can be confused with the development of a lymphoma. Initially similar to glandular fever, symptoms include sore throat, swollen glands in the neck, armpits and groin, headache, fever, night sweats and generalised skeletal and muscular aches. A feeling of extreme exhaustion is also reported. Distorted vision, sight loss, irregular or rapid heartbeat, loss of appetite and weight, skin and gum lesions and excessive thirst have also been reported. Some of these symptoms may be present all the time – others may only occur during a flare-up.

This can also be the pattern of infection in immunosuppressed patients, where there can either be a reactivation of an historic infection or a new infection. In HIV patients the development of clinical toxoplasmosis is one of the markers for transition to ARC. Reactivation can cause inflammatory lesions in the brain, leading to headache, impaired coordination, seizures, sensory loss, tremor, loss of vision, personality changes, disorientation and coma. Abscesses may also be present in the central nervous system. In a new infection, the disease is rapid and severe, requiring prompt and thorough therapeutic intervention.[30]

The pathogen may also cause severe pneumonitis, and can affect the retina with consequent loss of vision, and ultimately blindness.

Diagnosis

Diagnosis in pregnant women is usually made using pathogen-specific antibody testing of blood samples. Any positive findings are confirmed by a *Toxoplasma* reference unit.

Polymerase chain reaction (PCR) tests on tissue and fluid samples have also been used; at present there is no commercially available test. In AIDS/HIV patients antibody testing is not considered useful, as it only confirms that exposure has occurred, and as many cases are the results of reactivation of dormant cysts, other methods are needed to determine the status of the individual in relation to infection or active disease. Biopsy specimens of brain tissue can detect cysts, and the presence of tachyzoites is a sign of active disease.

Computerised tomography, magnetic resonance imaging and

radiographic imaging can also be used to detect cysts in the central nervous system, and monitor the effectiveness of therapeutic interventions.

Treatment

For most cases of toxoplasmosis, no therapeutic intervention is required. For pregnant women, HIV/AIDS sufferers and any individual with optical involvement, intervention is necessary. Treatment is particularly essential where evidence of encephalitis is seen. The *BNF*[13] recommends a combination of pyrimethamine and sulfadiazine given for a period of weeks, with addition of folinic acid if required. Combinations of pyrimethamine and clindamycin or azithromycin or clarithromycin have also been used. Expert advice is essential when drug therapy is initiated, and with the toxicity of the agents used, constant monitoring is required, as pyrimethamine is a folate antagonist. Spiramycin, widely used in continental Europe for toxoplasmosis treatment, is available in the UK on a named-patient basis from IDIS Ltd, and may reduce the risk of transmission of maternal infection to the fetus. Steroids are used as an adjunctive therapy to reduce intracranial pressure.

It must be borne in mind that although the condition will respond to treatment, long-term therapy is necessary to prevent recurrence, and monitoring is essential. Individuals who have survived toxoplasmosis encephalitis (TE) should have lifelong prophylaxis. In some studies into the effectiveness of post-TE prophylaxis relapse rates of between 20% and 30% have been seen. Non-compliance is a major problem, and relates to the complexity of dosing needed, as is the spectrum of adverse events associated with long-term use of these therapeutic moieties.

In the USA, a different regime is used for both prevention and treatment of toxoplasmosis in HIV/AIDS patients. Trimethoprim and sulfamethoxazole (co-trimoxazole) is used to prevent both TE and *Pneumocystis carinii* pneumonia (PCP). In patients who cannot tolerate this drug combination, dapsone and pyrimethamine are used; again, this combination is effective against TE and PCP. Folinic acid is added to all these regimes. Atovaquone, with or without pyrimethamine, has also been used with some success. Dosage regimens vary depending upon complicating factors – including pregnancy – and adverse reactions, response to therapy, and age or weight of the subject.

When to commence therapy and monitoring and decisions on duration of therapy should be made by specialist units or consultants. Specific dosages are not given, as regimes change and alter rapidly with new research and trials being carried out.

Prevention

It is recommended that all individuals in high-risk groups eat only meat that has been thoroughly cooked, and avoid consuming raw cured meats such as Parma ham or cured venison. Unpasteurised goat's or ewe's milk and cheese should not be eaten. Good food hygiene should be routine: all fruit and vegetables should be washed before being eaten and all utensils should be washed well after raw meat has been processed. Personal hygiene routines and hand-washing should be as frequent as necessary to prevent infection. Gloves should be worn when cleaning cat litter trays. This should be undertaken daily to remove the infective focus before any oocysts shed in the faecal matter can mature to an infectious stage. In HIV/AIDS patients it may be preferable for another person, who is not in a high-risk group, to carry out tray cleaning.[29]

Children should be encouraged in good personal hygiene habits, and wherever possible sandpits and other areas should be covered when not in use and cleaned to remove feline faecal material promptly. Patients in at-risk groups should wear gloves when gardening and clean both hands and gloves after use.

Pet cats belonging to people in at-risk groups should be kept inside and fed canned or dry foods to prevent infection from wild rodents or undercooked meat. Provided adequate precautions are undertaken, there is no need to remove the cat from the domestic scene permanently.

Sheep may be inoculated against toxoplasmosis. This carries some risk to the operatives involved, and they should rapidly seek medical advice if accidental inoculation occurs.

Useful addresses

Toxoplasmosis Trust
61–71 Collier Street
London N1 9BE

Tommy's Campaign have now taken over the work of the Toxoplasmosis Trust. However the Toxoplasmosis Trust website, www.toxo.org.uk, still offers useful fact sheets for healthcare workers and patients.

Tommy's Campaign
1 Kennington Road
London SE1 7RR
Tel: +44 (0)20 7620 0188
www.tommys-campaign.org

Dogs

Introduction

The PFMA survey for 2000 shows an estimated 6.5 million dogs in 5.1 million households across the UK. Whilst the population of cats has increased over the last decade, so the number of dogs has shown a steady decline. The same pressures of work and housing have caused the more dependent canine to lose some of its place at the hearth side.

However, dogs are not just kept as companions; working dogs are still part of the farming enterprise, and the sheepdog is still invaluable for managing sheep, especially on extensive upland farms. Dogs are also used by the police, and as drug and explosive detectors, not forgetting hearing dogs for the deaf and guide dogs for the blind.

The particular and peculiar bond between dogs and humans is ancient, and the recognition of the risks involved in close contact with canines is well documented. At present the UK remains rabies-free, and with vigilance and care this most dramatic of canine-carried zoonotic diseases should continue to be excluded.

Many of the zoonoses associated with cats may also be seen in dogs, although the pathogen responsible may be species-specific. The zoonosis in this section is particularly dramatic and arises out of the very specific bond of the sheepdog to both sheep and humans in its labours.

Other zoonoses associated with dogs may be found by referring to the index.

Echinoccosis
(Unilocular hydatid disease or hydatidosis)

Worldwide, echinoccosis is caused by two species of tapeworm, *Echinococcus granulosus*, and *E. multilocularis*. They belong to a sub-group of tapeworms known as tissue cestodes, as for part of their life cycle they encyst in body tissues. In the UK only *E. granulosus* has been found; *E. multilocularis* is seen in other countries in western Europe. Elsewhere in the world both organisms are seen over a wide geographical range. The disease associated with *E. granulosus* is known as unilocular hydatid, as only a single site is initially colonised, whereas *E. multilocularis* colonises multiple sites simultaneously and therefore leads to more serious clinical disease. There is a theoretical risk that tourists or travellers could pick up *E. multilocularis* whilst abroad. In the UK cases are usually confined to areas where there is intensive sheep farming, especially in mid-Wales, Hereford and Scotland.

In humans these tapeworms cause a condition known as hydatid disease where cysts of great size may develop over long periods post-infection (Plate 3). Luckily, human infections in the UK with the tapeworm larvae responsible for the condition are rare. Over the last decade there has been reporting of between 5 and 26 cases annually, although it would appear that reporting is incomplete. As the disease has a long prepatent period of between 10 and 20 years before cysts become palpable, the numbers of people with the disease may be higher since many subclinical cases may go undetected where there is no autopsy following death from other causes.

Disease in animals

These species of tapeworm require both dogs (and foxes) and sheep to be present in the same environment for their complete normal life cycle to take place. Humans, although they can suffer the unpleasant effects of infection by these organisms, are a dead-end host in which the tapeworm cannot complete the cycle (Figure 2.4). In the UK, sheep are the most important intermediate host, although cattle, horses and pigs can also carry the encysted larval stage.

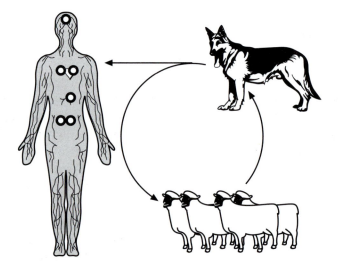

Figure 2.4 Hydatidosis in humans and the life cycle of *Echinococcus granulosus* in dogs and sheep. Open circles show likely sites for hydatid cyst formation.

The normal life cycle of the tapeworm consists of the following phases: a sheep grazing on contaminated pastures ingests eggs in faecal matter from dogs or foxes. The sheep acts as the intermediate host and after ingestion the eggs hatch into larvae which migrate through the intestinal wall and then encyst in the organs and tissues. After death, dogs eat tissue from the sheep contaminated with cysts and after ingestion the encysted larvae emerge and progress to adult tapeworms in the intestine of the dog. Eggs are then produced and pass out with the faecal matter, and so the cycle commences once more.

In animals infection is often asymptomatic, although a heavy burden of developing larvae or adult worms may lead to diarrhoea. In dogs, segments of the adult worm or even the worm may become apparent either in the stools or in some cases protruding from the anus. Inspection of meat from inspected sheep after slaughter can detect cysts. Such carcasses will be condemned for human or animal consumption.

Transmission

Human infection follows consumption of food or water contaminated with viable eggs from dog faeces. In the USA there is some evidence that infection may also occur by a hand-to-mouth route after stroking a dog with faecal contamination, or by handling objects contaminated with faecal matter.

Disease in humans

Following infection, the eggs hatch and the resulting larvae migrate and then encyst. The encysted larvae will then commence a slow growth and multiplication process to form multiple hydatids, an infective larval form. Known as hydatid sand, this may consist of thousands of particles in a large cyst. Due to the slow growth, physical detection of the cyst may only follow after more than a decade. The most common site where the cyst forms is in the liver, with the mass restricted by a thickened membrane. Clinical signs and detection follow abdominal swelling and pressure on other internal organs or bile duct obstruction with associated nausea and pain. The retaining membrane may rupture into the abdomen, pericardium or pleural cavity with the possibility of anaphylactic shock or severe allergic response to the fluid contained within the cyst or the hydatid particles. Death may follow, as can the formation of new cysts in other locations by the released hydatids.

Primary cysts may also form in other sites, with the lungs, kidneys, central nervous system and bone marrow being in decreasing order the most likely sites. Lung cysts are usually asymptomatic until they become large enough to block airways or they rupture. Persistent dry cough, pain or coughing blood may occur. Cysts in the central nervous system cause symptoms earlier than those in other locations, with epileptiform fits or paraesthesia. Spontaneous fracture and bone pain can be a result of cysts in the bone marrow, with the most common sites being the vertebrae. Compression of the spinal cord or dependent nerves may follow, with associated paralysis or weakness.

Diagnosis

Diagnosis is usually made by radiography or serology testing. Exploratory or investigative surgery can be risky unless precautions are taken to avoid membrane rupture.

Treatment

Treatment traditionally was surgical to remove the cyst or cysts and the contents. Postsurgery washing-out of the affected body cavity with ethanol, formaldehyde solution, hypertonic saline, iodine solution, hydrogen peroxide or silver nitrate solution has been recommended to destroy any hydatids which have escaped the cyst membrane, and which could begin new cysts. Although surgery is still seen as the main option, the BNF[13] recommends adjunctive use of albendazole (available from IDIS Ltd on a named-patient basis under the trade name Zentel) to prevent formation of secondary foci or in inoperable cases.[31] Dual therapy with cimetidine and mebendazole has also been trialled, with addition of the cimetidine to increase blood levels of the anthelmintic.[32, 33] In the USA praziquantel has also been used as a treatment both as a mono-therapy and as an adjunct to surgery. There is some evidence for the use of albendazole and praziquantel in combination for postoperative treatment as there are some doubts expressed as to the efficiency of single agents, especially long-term.[34]

The WHO recommends albendazole 800 mg/day in divided doses for 28 days, followed by 14 drug-free days as a treatment cycle. Where surgery is impossible, the WHO suggests repeat treatments for up to three full cycles. As an adjunct in surgical treatment of hydatid cysts, pre- and/or postsurgery, one cycle is suggested.

Prevention

Prevention strategies include the regular worming of dogs, especially working sheepdogs with praziquantel (Droncit: Bayer). Stray dogs should be controlled by the usual methods of impounding or culling. Feeding dogs with sheep offal or infected meat should be avoided, with rigorous abattoir checks to prevent infected meat entering the food chain. Preventing human infection, as with other parasitic diseases such as *Toxoplasma*, relates to implementation of strict hygiene measures and education. The condition is considered to be an occupational hazard for shepherds and others who work with sheep.

Although cases of echinoccosis associated with *E. multilocularis* have never been confirmed in the UK, a few notes are appended for the sake of completeness. Infection with *E. multilocularis*, also known as alveolar disease, follows the same pattern, with ingestion of eggs associated with faecal contamination from dogs, cats or foxes. The normal intermediate hosts are rodents rather than sheep. The cycle is completed when dogs, cats or foxes eat mice or other infected rodents. Unlike cysts associated with *E. granulosus* the cysts of *E. multilocularis* have no membrane and can therefore spread from the original foci more rapidly. Primary foci are usually in liver or lungs and occasionally in other tissue sites. The associated hydatids are invasive and the condition can be rapidly fatal, with an estimated 90% of untreated cases dying within 10 years.

Horses

Introduction

According to a survey carried out by the British Horse Society in 1999 (available at http://www.bhs.org.uk), there were 900 000 horses in the UK, from shetlands to shires, via hunters, to cobs and racehorses. Approximately 2.4 million people ride, some occasionally, but many routinely as part of their lifestyle or work.

Horses and their riders participate in many events, from the Horse of the Year show, to the local gymkhana, and keeping horses as a leisure activity is becoming ever more popular. With this amount of human–animal contact, there is always some risk of medical problems. Luckily there are few zoonoses solely carried by equines; the likelihood of injury from other horse-associated activities is greater, with falls, kicks and occasional bites requiring the most acute medical care.

The diseases discussed in this section are, or have been, of major significance. Glanders was feared until the beginning of the last century, and has re-emerged as a significant zoonosis in other areas of the world. With the flooding that much of the country has experienced in recent years, the incidence of leptospirosis is increasing and is likely to become more significant in future if the changes in weather patterns are sustained.

Tetanus is still a major issue in terms of public health measures, and the control of the disease requires constant application of a comprehensive vaccination programme.

Horses can transmit or carry other zoonotic diseases which are normally primarily associated with other animals. This is mentioned in other sections under the primary host animal. References to these conditions will be found in the index.

Glanders, farcy and melioidosis

Glanders or farcy is caused by the bacterium *Burkholderia* (formerly *Pseudomonas*) *mallei*. It is a notifiable disease of especially horses but also donkeys and mules. Goats, cats and dogs have also been known to acquire the disease. Import of susceptible animals from countries where the disease has been reported is forbidden. Recently DEFRA issued a notice to that effect relating to horses from Brazil after an outbreak there. Geographically, the disease is endemic in Africa, Asia, the Middle East and Central and South America.

Melioidosis, also called Whitmore's disease, is clinically and pathologically similar to glanders and is caused by the same organism. It is predominantly a disease of tropical climates, especially in South-east Asia where it is endemic. The disease is contracted from contaminated water and soil and is spread to humans and animals through direct contact with the contaminated source. Melioidosis is not considered to be a zoonosis, although the animal population in endemic areas forms the infective reservoir. Glanders is a zoonosis, as humans contract the disease from infected domestic animals.[35]

Individuals who contract this disease as a result of their work are entitled to compensation payments under Social Security rules. It is considered under the provisions of the Health and Safety at Work Act and also as a prescribed disease by the Industrial Injuries Advisory Council. The last recorded case in the UK occurred in 1928, but it is possible that many subclinical cases are not seen or identified due to blind antibiotic use without sample culture.

Historically it was very significant as it causes rapid fatality in horses and humans – this was a disaster in a society which was reliant on true horsepower for its transport of both people and goods. In 1902 many London boroughs closed their public animal water troughs because of an outbreak of the disease. In human patients in the era before antimicrobial agents were available, 95% of victims with clinical signs would die. The use of antibiotics has reduced this toll dramatically.

Human infection is luckily now rare; however, it has been seen in pulmonary (glanders) and cutaneous (farcy) forms. It can affect stable personnel or people in close physical contact with horses in the course of their work. Infection in laboratory workers has also been seen. The inoculum necessary to cause infection is small, and the organism has been considered as a potential agent for biological warfare or terrorism.[36]

Transmission

The organism is spread by discharge from wounds and aerosols. Ingestion, inhalation or physical contact with the inoculum allows the bacterium to colonise the next victim. In several cases the initial inoculum has also occurred through the eye or nasal mucosa. Physical inoculation of wounds or abrasions with infected material has been shown to occur. In melioidosis sexual transfer has been demonstrated and there is a single report of this also occurring in farcy, where human-to-human spread occurred. Once across the species barrier, patients' carers, especially where there is close physical contact, are at risk.

Disease in humans

Following inoculation, the incubation period usually ranges from 1–14 days. Symptoms in humans are dependent on the route of transmission. The cutaneous form is characterised by skin pustules which suppurate; localised lymph node swelling may then occur. Non-specific symptoms can include headache, with raised temperature, and aching muscles. If mucosal membranes are involved, excessive tear production or nasal discharge may be seen. The disease can then become systemic with an undulant fever, enlargement of the liver and spleen, an overwhelming septicaemia and a high associated mortality rate if left untreated.

The pulmonary form follows the same pattern in terms of early non-specific symptoms; subsequently pneumonia develops with copious mucus production. Abscess formation in the lung may occur with pleurisy and lung collapse.

The bacteria may be shed in urine, blood, mucosal secretions and in the pus from skin lesions, leading to a risk of further infection.

Treatment

Human cases of glanders are rare so limited information is available about antibiotic treatment of the organism in humans. This also leads to problems with diagnosis, as serological assays are not reliable or readily available. Culturing the organism is time-consuming and, as the disease can be rapidly fatal, treatment usually commences on the presumption of illness.

Sulfadiazine at a dose of 25 mg/kg intravenously four times a day has been found to be effective in experimental animals and in humans. *B. mallei* is also usually sensitive to some or all of the following: penicillins (particularly amoxicillin either alone or in combination as co-amoxiclav), tetracyclines (especially doxycycline), ciprofloxacin, streptomycin, gentamicin, ticarcillin, azlocillin, imipenem, aztreonam, ceftazidime and ceftriaxone. Resistance to chloramphenicol has been reported. Streptomycin in combination with tetracyclines or chloramphenicol has been used historically in the USA but has been replaced by other agents. Where systemic infection with deep-tissue abscesses is present, therapy may have to be prolonged to resolve the infection: durations of more than 14 days have been reported.[37]

Prevention

No vaccine is available to prevent infection with *B. mallei*. Where the infection is endemic, prevention strategies consist of controlling and eliminating the disease in the animal reservoir. Any patient suspected of being infected must be carefully nursed to avoid infection, with appropriate measures including gloves, masks and gowns.

Leptospirosis
*(Weil's disease, haemorrhagic jaundice (*Leptospira icterohaemorrhagiae*), canicola fever (*L. canicola*), dairy-worker fever (*L. hardjo*))*

Leptospirosis is caused by motile spirochaetes of the genus *Leptospira*. These organisms occur worldwide and are most common in temperate or tropical climates. They may be found associated with animals and humans, or free-living in water or soil. The particular organism responsible for a variety of potentially zoonotic infections is *L. interrogans*, of which there are more than 200 serotypes; each is species-specific. The most important are *L. hardjo*, associated with cattle and horses, *L. icterohaemorrhagiae*, found in rodents and dogs (specifically the organism responsible for Weil's disease), *L. canicola* in dogs, and *L. pomona* in pigs and cattle. Incidence of the disease ranges from endemic in some areas to sporadic in others. More cases are seen in areas that have been flooded, as soil-living pathogens are released into the surface water and cause wider contamination of potable water sources.

The disease is notifiable under the Public Health (Infectious Diseases) Regulations 1988. It is considered by the HSE to be a hazard at work and is subject to the Control of Substances Hazardous to Health (COSHH) regulations 1994 in terms of provision of protective clothing and prevention measures for persons at risk of occupational exposure. The disease is also covered by Reporting of Injuries, Diseases, and Dangerous Occurrences Regulations (RIDDOR).

Disease in animals

The pattern of clinical signs in infected animals varies from species to species. Cattle often present with weight loss and a high fever, with mastitis in 'in-milk' heifers and declining milk yields. This disease is the most frequently diagnosed cause of bovine abortion in the UK: abortion occurs spontaneously in 'in-calf' heifers with afterbirth retention. Hepatic enlargement, anaemia and jaundice may also be seen. In dogs, acute haemorrhage, jaundice and hepatitis are seen with infection with *L. canicola*, and kidney damage in infection with *L. icterohaemorrhagiae*. Diarrhoea and gastritis may also be seen. Rodents are the only genus which can show no sign of disease, yet are able to shed viable organisms throughout their lives, and are considered to be not only a reservoir for the disease, but also a vector. Organisms are shed in the urine of infected animals and contaminate soil or water.

Transmission

Transmission to humans usually follows either ingestion of water contaminated with infected animal urine, and particularly that of rodents, or contact with contaminated soil or food. The organism can also enter the body by skin abrasions or cuts, and also via the mucosal membranes of the nose, mouth or eyes. Bathing or swimming in infected waters appears to be a major route. The disease is an occupational hazard for sewage, water and canal workers. Vets, aid workers and watersport enthusiasts are also at a higher than average risk of contracting the disease. There are no recorded incidents of human-to-human transfer. There were 29 confirmed reports of leptospirosis in humans during 1998, of which *L. icterohaemorrhagiae* and *L. hardjo* both caused nine each. The other 11 were the result of other serotypes. There is believed to be massive underreporting of cases.[38]

Disease in humans

Following infection, there is a prepatent period ranging from a few days to several weeks. Clinical signs vary from inapparent to severe acute manifestations with associated mortality. The onset may be sudden with high fever, headaches, aching muscles and joints and fatigue. Vomiting may occur, and hepatic enlargement with associated jaundice is common. Depending upon the causative organism and the severity of the disease there may be a second phase of the disease. After an apparent recovery the patient becomes ill again with declining kidney and liver function, mental confusion and delusion, meningitis, breathing difficulties and catastrophic hypotension. In the second phase, symptoms are continuous and do not regress until recovery or death occurs. This biphasic form is associated with *L. icterohaemorrhagiae* and is known as Weil's disease or icteric leptospirosis, although it only occurs in approximately one-tenth of patients infected in any outbreak. The disease may last for days or weeks and untreated it carries a risk of 5–10% case mortality rate. Recovery can be prolonged, with an extended convalescence of months after clinical illness ends.

Many of the symptoms of the disease can be mistaken for other diseases (for instance, dengue fever, malaria and typhus), so differential diagnosis may be difficult. Nevertheless, diagnosis is of paramount importance to allow treatment to commence quickly. Rapid treatment is essential to prevent progression and associated mortality.

Diagnosis

Early in the disease, the organism may be identified by dark-field microscopy of a blood film or by culture. The organism is difficult to grow on conventional media and may require a period of weeks to establish identifiable colonies. More rapid diagnosis can be made using a dot-enzyme-linked immunosorbent assay (DOT-ELISA) test. Recently a dip test stick has been developed using an immunoglobulin agglutination method by the Centers for Disease Control and Prevention in the

USA. This has allowed rapid diagnosis and enables early therapeutic intervention.

Treatment

Treatment is normally with penicillin at normal therapeutic doses or, in the case of penicillin allergy, tetracyclines at normal doses as alternative drugs of choice. Therapy should be initiated early in the course of disease and intravenous antibiotics should be used for persons with severe manifestations.

Studies carried out in the USA suggest that prophylaxis using oral doxycycline at a dose of 200 mg/week is effective in reducing infection in groups at high risk, either due to their occupational or recreational pursuits.

Prevention

In the UK, dogs and cattle may be vaccinated against the disease, reducing the infective reservoir. The vaccination is not necessarily routine in cattle as vaccinated cattle may be unacceptable for export to certain countries.

Wherever possible individuals should avoid swimming in or drinking from potentially contaminated water. Workers likely to suffer occupational exposure should be supplied with adequate protective clothing. Rodent populations must be controlled wherever possible and prophylaxis with antibiotics should be considered for workers, especially where cases have been reported. Rodent carcasses should not be handled and cuts and abrasions should be covered with plasters or dressings.[39]

Tetanus

Caused by *Clostridium tetani*, a typical anaerobic spore-forming Gram-positive bacterium of the *Clostridium* group, tetanus was well known as a major cause of fatality following traumatic injury. The bacterium is found fairly universally in the environment. It is capable of multiplying in the guts of animals, often without causing clinical disease. It is then passed in the faeces and forms spores in large numbers in dung. Ground or equipment contaminated with dung or animal manure can act as a focus for infection. In folklore, the disease was always associated with horses and stables, although there is no proof that equines are more prolific amplifiers of the organism than other mammals.

Spores of *C. tetani* are very persistent, and are capable of remaining viable for long periods. Tetanus was a recognised risk in agriculture and also warfare, with many of the soldiers 'succumbing to their wounds' dying as a result of tetanus. In the late 1880s, the organism was identified and isolated, and production of the first antitoxin followed in the next decade. By the beginning of the First World War the use of passive immunisation was routine, both as treatment and prophylaxis. By the onset of the Second World War a more sophisticated regime of tetanus toxoid and attenuated active immunisation was made available.

The disease can be fatal, and is still a major cause of death in developing countries, where immunisation programmes are inadequate, or where the uptake rate of vaccination is low. Neonates and children are particularly at risk, as are the elderly. Neonate tetanus following dressing of the umbilicus with cattle dung has decreased as this practice has become less prevalent. There are estimated to be about one million clinical cases worldwide each year.[40]

Disease in animals

The organism does not affect most healthy animals and they tend to develop immunity rapidly, although there may be fatalities especially in neonates. The disease normally commences after traumatic wounds are infected and leads to muscle spasm and respiratory difficulty, resulting in death.

Disease in humans

Owing to the high level of immunisation in the UK – nearly 96% in 1999 – fewer than 100 clinical cases are reported each year. Cases are normally seen in individuals who have either never received vaccination, or who have neglected their booster injections. In the USA an identified high-risk group is injecting heroin addicts. Heroin which has been cut with brick dust or admixtured with quinine can lead to disease. It is believed that the quinine can increase the rate at which the bacteria multiply after inoculation. An interesting comparison can be found in the case history on gas gangrene (see p. 74).[41]

Infection follows deep, penetrating wounds or severe surface abrasions with inadequate cleaning procedures, especially in tissues or structures where there is poor perfusion and low oxygenation. Wounds from high-velocity objects such as bullets and shrapnel fragments, as well as stab wounds, burns or frostbite, are particularly associated with clinical cases of this disease. Minor wounds which are ignored or neglected can also pose a risk. Thorough cleansing and debridement are essential in good wound care, and are particularly crucial where the risk of tetanus is high.[42]

After infection the spores rapidly become transformed into active bacteria. The prepatent period can vary from a few days to several months. The first clinical signs are generalised: the patient complains of headache and irritability with muscular weakness, cramping or stiffening. There may be difficulty in chewing and swallowing.

As the bacteria continue to multiply they release an exotoxin. In about 80% of cases the disease presents as generalised tetanus. This affects the motor neurons and the central nervous system. Overstimulation of the motor neurons follows and painful, prolonged contractions of muscle and spasm occur progressively. The spasm usually commences in the face, producing a condition known as trismus or lockjaw. The spasm produces a rigid expression (*risus sardonicus* – literally, 'the sardonic smile'). Spread to other muscle groups follows, with spasm in the back and limbs. Seizures may occur. The contractions of the muscles may be severe enough to cause bone fractures. Spasms occur frequently and last for a period of minutes. The intercostal muscles in the ribcage are affected and breathing may become difficult, requiring external support. Heart rate rises, due to neural damage or block, and hypertension occurs. In untreated cases, exhaustion and respiratory failure lead on to death.

The other two forms of the disease are local tetanus and cephalic tetanus. Local tetanus consists of spasm solely in the limb nearest to the original inoculation site; the condition may last for weeks and can progress to generalised tetanus. Cephalic tetanus usually follows middle-ear infections or head injury. The cranial nerves become involved rapidly, and the facial nerves are worst affected.

Access to intensive care facilities with mechanical ventilators has decreased fatalities; however, case rate fatality is usually about 30% despite treatment, depending upon the pattern and progress of the disease. Recovery can be prolonged. Muscle spasm slowly regresses after about 10–14 days, but full return to normal function is slow and residual damage may persist for many months or years. Many fatalities result from secondary infections of the lungs or other organs by opportunistic pathogens. Heart failure or stroke may further complicate the clinical course of disease and treatment.

Treatment

Where a patient has tetanic muscle spasm the *BNF*[13] recommends the use of diazepam intravenously at a dose of 100–300 µg/kg repeated every 1–4 hours as needed. The same drug can also be administered by intravenous infusion or by nasoduodenal tube at a rate of 3–10 mg/kg over 24 hours, adjusting the dose according to response. Chlorpromazine has been used to reduce spasm in severe established cases.

The *BNF*[13] also states that benzylpenicillin (penicillin G) is effective when used in the treatment of tetanus, although it has now been replaced by metronidazole as the preferred drug. In established cases metronidazole is given by intravenous infusion at a rate of 500 mg every 8 hours in adults, and at a rate of 7.5 mg/kg every 8 hours in children.

Any patient in whom tetanus is suspected and who has an incomplete immunisation history or established infection should receive human tetanus immunoglobulin (HTIG) as soon as possible. This binds any free toxin before it can attach to neural receptors, but it does not destroy any toxin already bound. Recommended doses vary depending on the manufacturer's data. Careful study of the guidance in the *BNF* should be made before administration. As a guide, a dose of 250 units should be given intramuscularly, doubled to 500 units where longer than 12–24 hours has elapsed since injury or where heavy infection is likely. Special recommendations are in place for immunocompromised individuals, or other patients in whom standard immunisation regimes cannot be used. Suspected cases which fall into these groups are best treated by specialist centres. HTIG may also be used in established cases at a rate of 150 units/kg using multiple injection sites. Intravenous HTIG at a rate of 5000–10 000 units is also used in proven or suspected clinical cases.

Prevention

Tetanus exotoxin is not antigenic, and infection does not usually confer immunity. Immunisation is the most important measure in preventing the disease. Children normally receive tetanus vaccine as part of the triple vaccine programme, and subsequent booster doses within the childhood vaccine confer the necessary immunity. A further booster using adsorbed tetanus vaccine (sometimes referred to as tetanus toxoid) should be given at intervals of 10 years. Adsorbed vaccine can also be used in a course of three injections at 4-week intervals to produce immunity in individuals in whom either primary vaccination has not occurred, or where longer than 10 years has elapsed since the last dose. Any adult who has had five or more doses of vaccine is likely to have acquired lifelong immunity.

Wound care is also important in preventing infection, and appropriate measures should be taken to clean all wounds thoroughly as soon as possible.

Gas gangrene

Clostridial gas gangrene can be produced by at least six different species of *Clostridium*. *C. perfringens* (previously known as *C. welchii*) is responsible for most cases, but *C. novyi*, *C. septicum* and *C. chauvoei* are also significant causative organisms for this condition. More than one species of *Clostridium* may be present during the course of the infection. Gas gangrene carries a high level of mortality. Before antibiotics were readily available and effective as treatment, the only therapeutic intervention available was amputation. In established clinical cases mortality even after treatment can be as high as 30%. All untreated cases are rapidly fatal.[43]

C. perfringens, *C. novyi* and *C. chauvoei* are found in pigs, sheep and cattle. They may be amplified by animals and are normal gut inhabitants. They are passed in the faeces and, as with *C. tetani*, can become environmental contaminants, especially on pasture and areas contaminated with dung.

Disease in animals

Each of the clostridia considered here causes a slightly different clinical disease. They are, however, also very similar in the way the disease develops.

C. perfringens can cause two different diseases in sheep depending on the serotype of the pathogen. Pulpy kidney or enterotoxaemia is associated with type D. Clinical disease follows the rapid multiplication of this pathogen in the gut, where it forms part of the normal flora. The rapid multiplication produces significant amounts of exotoxin which, following absorption through the intestinal wall, causes sudden death with cardiac damage and internal haemorrhage. Lamb dysentery is often caused by *C. perfringens* type B. It affects lambs usually within a week of birth in endemic areas, with blood-stained diarrhoea causing rapid fluid loss and fatal dehydration and haemorrhage. On autopsy the gut is found to be ulcerated and may be perforated. The same organism is also responsible for a similar condition in pigs called pigbel, where destruction of the gut follows release of exotoxin. This condition is covered in Chapter 4.

This group of bacteria are also responsible for several other animal diseases. *C. perfringens* type B causes a condition colloquially known as struck, and follows the same pattern of infection, colonisation, exotoxin production and death. *C. septicum* is responsible for a similar condition known as braxy, which follows colonisation and destruction of portions of the sheep's rumen.

C. chauvoei causes a condition known as black quarter. This affliction follows a very similar course to gas gangrene in humans, and *C. septicum* may also be present. Following inoculation into a deep penetrating wound, usually in the leg, the pathogen causes tissue necrosis and gas production. Progress of the disease is rapid: the infected tissue becomes black and ruptures as quantities of gas are produced in the dead tissue. Exotoxin production causes rapid death. The same organism can also cause a condition designated gangrenous metritis in postpartum ewes, where the uterus is colonised and invasion of tissue and exotoxin production occur, with the loss of the ewe. The condition may also affect young cattle.

Disease in humans

Infection usually follows inoculation of deep wounds in poorly perfused muscle tissue as a result of traumatic injury, although the condition can result from rupture of the intestinal tract in association with certain cancers or other conditions.[44] Field or amateur surgery, traumatic fractures, frostbite, burns, drug abuse and immunosuppression can also predispose patients to the condition. The ultimate outcome of the infection depends upon the site of injury – wounds in the limbs carry less risk of death than those in the trunk. In spontaneous cases where the infection is a result of gut trauma there is a 67–100% fatality rate.

There is a prepatent period of between 12 and 24 hours, although in the case of large inocula, clinical symptoms may be seen within 1 hour. The wound becomes painful and in the area around the wound a very slight inflammation may be present. The skin becomes shiny, gradually darkening and turning a brown or bronze colour. The area becomes tender to the touch and discharge occurs from the original wound. This discharge is copious and has an unpleasant sweet odour, sometimes described as 'mousy'. Once smelt, it is an odour that is always recognisable.

The mechanism of disease progression relates to exotoxin production and colonisation by the pathogen(s). *C. perfringens* is able to produce a mixture of exotoxins, including several enzymes. Kappatoxin can destroy connective tissue, and alphatoxin destroys erythrocytes and platelets, triggering histamine production, clotting and thrombosis. The resulting necrosis produced by the onslaught of the exotoxins can spread at a rate of 2 cm/h. There is slowing of the heart rate and breathing, with a fall in blood pressure. The patient may become cyanosed with symptoms of toxic shock, kidney and liver failure. Death may follow within 12 hours in rapidly progressing cases.

Diagnosis

Diagnosis is usually presumptive, although microscopy of tissue or exudate and neuraminidase tests are used as confirmation. Culturing the organism is not a viable option, as the patient will probably die before identification is possible. Bubbles of gas may be detected in tissue using X-ray images.

Treatment

Once a diagnosis is made or presumed, treatment must be initiated as soon as possible. The *BNF*[13] recommends the use of penicillin G in adults at a rate of 1.2 g/day by intramuscular or slow intravenous injection or infusion, increasing in adults up to 2.4 g/day in divided doses, or more if the situation warrants it. Paediatric dosages start at 100 mg/kg daily in four divided doses, and may be increased if needed.

American references mention the use of clindamycin at a dose of 600–1200 mg/day in divided 8-hourly doses intravenously, or 20–40 mg/kg daily in children, also intravenously in divided 8-hourly doses. The main hazard is considered to be hepatic insufficiency. Chloramphenicol and metronidazole have also been used.

In all cases the hazards associated with the antibiotic therapy at high doses pale into insignificance beside the risks of the condition.

Hyperbaric oxygen therapy is recommended wherever possible in conjunction with antibiotics. If available, it should be introduced as soon as diagnosis is made, whether confirmed or not. The use of oxygen reduces the ability of the pathogen to reproduce, and also to survive or produce the exotoxins responsible for tissue damage. Oxygen has been used successfully in two regimes either three times normal atmospheric pressure for 90 minutes three times a day for 1 or 2 days, followed by the same treatment twice daily until the disease is controlled, or 2.5 times atmospheric pressure for 2 hours in the same regime of daily repeats. The use of oxygen therapy may reduce or remove the need for amputation; however, the wound may need to be surgically opened to allow the oxygen to penetrate.[45]

Surgical intervention with active debridement of wounds to remove necrotic tissue as an adjunct to other therapies is essential. If amputation must be undertaken, it often has to be radical.

Prevention

The *BNF*[13] recommends the use of benzylpenicillin at a rate of 300–600 mg by intramuscular or slow intravenous infusion every 6 hours for 5 days, or metronidazole 500 mg every 8 hours by intravenous infusion, as antibiotic prophylaxis in high lower-limb amputations or following major traumatic wounds.

Vaccination is the preferred method of prevention for these diseases in animals. Some of the vaccines are solely for one condition, while others cover several diseases in combination. Antitoxins are also available. Their use is routine in sheep to prevent massive economic losses. Good hygiene practice at shearing and when lambs are having their tails docked or male lambs are castrated, prevents infection.

Case history

Contamination of a batch of street heroin with material containing the spores of *C. novyi* is believed to have been responsible for a number of deaths amongst addicts across the UK in the year 2000. More than 70 cases were reported across England, Scotland, Wales and Eire. Of the 36 fatalities associated with this incident, 18 occurred in Greater Glasgow.

All were injecting heroin users, and started to display symptoms of disease following accidental injection into muscle or soft tissue. Following injection, the addict could die within hours of multiple organ failure or after development of an abscess at the injection site; there could also be onset of gas gangrene.

It is possible that the citric acid used in preparing the drug before injection by the drug users increased the rate of development of the condition by activating the infective spores.[46]

Miscellaneous zoonoses of companion animals

All animals have diseases specific to species or genera. It is inevitable that some of the causative organisms of these diseases will be potential zoonoses. In general, the more unusual the animal, the more outrageous the possible zoonoses.

The fashion for keeping primates as pets has luckily almost disappeared as our closest cousins carry some very unpleasant pathogens. These may not cause clinical signs in the ape, but they are potentially fatal in humans. Apart from atypical mycobacteria and *Salmonella* spp., including *S. typhi*, simians can also harbour hepatitis A, herpes B virus (fatal in all recorded human cases), and other hazardous viruses such as Marburg (green monkey). Primates can also become aggressive as they mature. Bites or wounds inflicted on owners or keepers can rapidly become seriously infected and pose a serious hazard.

Reptiles such as turtles or terrapins, snakes and lizards have been identified as harbouring a variety of *Salmonella* spp. and are probably inappropriate as pets for owners who are not willing to become experts in their care and to devote sufficient time to appropriate hygiene routines.

There are many more zoonoses than it is possible to cover in a book of this size, and a decision has been made to exclude those which are not seen as being of major significance. As a final thought on the variety of pathogens which are potential zoonoses, it is enough to consider that armadillos are the only other known species in the world that can suffer from leprosy, apart from humans. No cases have ever been attributed to zoonotic spread, and nobody in the UK keeps armadillos as pets because their importation is prohibited under the Convention on International Trade in Endangered Species (CITES) treaty. This convention also controls trade in primates.

Notes to all case studies

These case studies aim to consolidate the knowledge gained from the text of this book. The case studies are brief and the questions are framed to encourage students to think around a condition or a risk group. This book was derived from material aimed at pharmacists, so some of the case studies are written from that standpoint. An attempt has been made to widen the horizon so that other professions will feel comfortable with the studies; however, temporarily other readers may have to become honorary pharmacy students and vice versa.

The answers are not prescriptive and may be found in Appendix 2. It is assumed that all the case studies relate to zoonotic infection of one type or another, but there may be other disease conditions, health issues or therapeutic solutions which are as appropriate as those found in the Case study answers section at the end of the book. Remember that this is a thinking and learning exercise, not a test with a pass mark.

CASE STUDIES

Case study 1

Mrs Carstairs, one of your elderly patients who lives alone, has had several bouts of chest infection with nasal discharge requiring repeated antibiotic therapy. She has also had two occurrences of conjunctivitis with persistent dry eyes. She mentions that Joey, her cockatoo, also seems to be 'under the weather' and losing condition along with his feathers.

Questions
1. Is it possible that the bird's condition and that of its mistress are related?
2. What might the condition be?
3. What should be the suggested action for either or both of the duo?

Case study 2

Miss Seymour is a lawyer and leads a very busy life. Her cats are her pride and joy: they are blue-point Persians of impeccable pedigree bred by her mother. The cats have the run of her flat and are allowed to sleep on her bed. She tells you she is having difficulties in seeing clearly, and this seems to have happened quite swiftly. She enquires if this could be a side-effect of the high-dose steroids she is currently taking for her asthma.

Questions
1. Could this be a side-effect of the therapy?
2. What zoonoses could produce this problem?
3. What action should she take?

References

1. Levits S M. The ecology of *Cryptococcus neoformans* and the epidemiology of cryptococcosis. *Rev Infect Dis* 1991; 3: 1163–1169.
2. Sánchez P, Bosch R J, de Gálvez M V, *et al*. Cutaneous cryptococcosis in two

patients with acquired immunodeficiency syndrome. *Int J STD AIDS* 2000; 11: 477–480.

3. Kim J H, Shin D H, Oh M D, *et al*. A case of disseminated cryptococcosis with skin eruption in a patient with acute leukemia scan. *J Infect Dis* 2001; 33: 234–235.

4. Belshe R B. Influenza as a zoonosis, how likely is a pandemic? *Lancet* 1998; 351: 460.

5. Bellingham C. Current issues in influenza. *Pharm J* 2001; 266: 57–59.

6. Taubenberger J K, Reid A H, Krafft A E, *et al*. Initial genetic characterization of the 1918 'Spanish' influenza virus. *Science* 1997; 275: 1793–1796.

7. Stuen S, Have P, Osterhaus A D, *et al*. Serological investigation of virus infections in harp seals (*groenlandica*) and hooded seals (*Cystophora cristata*). *Vet Rec* 1994; 134: 502–503.

8. Bradbury J. Hong Kong avian influenza characterised. *Lancet* 1998; 351: 189.

9. Dowdle W R. Pandemic influenza: confronting a re-emergent threat. The 1976 experience. *J Infect Dis* 1997; 176 (suppl. 1): S69–S72.

10. Hayden F G. Antivirals for pandemic influenza. *J Infect Dis* 1997; 176 (suppl. 1): S56–S61.

11. Prevention and control of influenza: recommendations of the Advisory Committee on Immunization Practices (ACIP). *MMWR* 1997; 46 (no. RR-9).

12. MAFF information sheets. *Animals and Animal Products (Import and Export) (England and Wales) Regulations*, 2000. *Products of Animal Origin (Import and Export) Regulations*, 1996. London: HMSO.

13. Mehta D K, ed. *British National Formulary*, vol. 42. London: British Medical Association/Royal Pharmaceutical Society of Great Britain, 2001.

14. Chaisson R E, Keiser P, Pierce M, *et al*. Clarithromycin and ethambutol with or without clofazimine for the treatment of bacteremic *Mycobacterium avium* complex disease in patients with HIV infection. *AIDS* 1997; 11: 311–317.

15. Havlir D V, Dube M P, Sattler F R, *et al*. Prophylaxis against disseminated *Mycobacterium avium* complex with weekly azithromycin, daily rifabutin, or both. *N Engl J Med* 1996; 335: 392–398.

16. Henry K, Crossley K. Wild-pigeon-related psittacosis in a family. *Chest* 1986; 90: 708–710.

17. Schaffner W. Birds of a feather – do they flock together? *Infect Control Hosp Epidemiol* 1997; 18: 162–164.

18. Bass J W, Vincent J M, Person D A. The expanding spectrum of *Bartonella* infections. II. Cat scratch disease. *Pediatr Infect Dis J* 1997; 16: 163–179.

19. Chomel B B. Cat scratch disease. *Rev Sci Tech* 2000; 19: 136–150.

20. Regnery R, Tappero J. Unraveling mysteries associated with cat-scratch disease, bacillary angiomatosis, and related syndromes. *Emerg Infect Dis* 1995; 1: 16–21.

21. Lowinger-Seoane M, Torres-Rodriguez J M, Madrenys-Brunet N, *et al*. Extensive dermatophytoses caused by *Trichophyton mentagrophytes* and *Microsporum canis* in a patient with AIDS. *Mycopathologia* 1992; 120: 143–146.

22. VandeWaa E A, Henderson J D, White G L, Nowatzke T J. Common

helminth infections: battling wormlike parasites in primary care. *Clin Rev* 1998; 8: 75–77, 81–82, 85–90, 92.

23. Lilley B, Lammie P, Dickerson J, Eberhard M. An increase in hookworm infection temporally associated with ecologic change. *Emerg Infect Dis* 1997; 3: 391–393.

24. DeSimone E M, Maag P. Common superficial fungal infections. *US Pharmacist* 1999; 24: online journal. http://www.uspharmacist.com

25. Hoff G L, Brawley J, Johnson K. Companion animal issues and the physician. *South Med J* 1999; 92: 651–659.

26. Glickman L T, Schantz P M. Epidemiology and pathogenesis of zoonotic toxocariasis. *Epidemiol Rev* 1981; 3: 230–250.

27. Kazacos K R. Visceral and ocular larva migrans. *Semin Vet Med Surg (Small Anim)* 1991; 6: 227–235.

28. Wallace M R, Rossetti R J, Olson P E. Cats and toxoplasmosis risk in HIV-infected adults. *JAMA* 1993; 269: 76–77.

29. Pham T S, Mansfield L S, Turiansky G W. Zoonoses in HIV-infected patients: risk factors and prevention. *AIDS Reader* 1997; 7: 41–52.

30. Flegr J, Zitkova S, Kodym P, Frynta D. Induction of changes in human behaviour by the parasitic protozoan *Toxoplasma gondii*. *Parasitology* 1996; 113: 49–54.

31. Nathan A. Anthelmintics. *Pharm J* 1997; 258: 770–771.

32. Bryceson A D, Cowie A G, Macleod C, *et al*. Experience with mebendazole in the treatment of inoperable hydatid disease in England. *Trans R Soc Trop Med Hyg* 1982; 76: 510–518.

33. Bekhti A, Pirotte J. Cimetidine increases serum mebendazole concentrations: implications for treatment of hepatic hydatid cysts. *Br J Clin Pharmacol* 1987; 24: 390–392.

34. Yasawy M I, Aal Karawi M A, Mohamed A R. Combination of praziquantel and albendazole in the treatment of hydatid disease. *Trop Med Parasitol* 1993; 44: 192–194.

35. Wilkinson L. Glanders: medicine and veterinary medicine in common pursuit of a contagious disease. *Med History* 1981; 25: 363–384.

36. Anonymous. Laboratory acquired human glanders. *MMWR* 2000; 49: 532–535.

37. Russell P, Eley S M, Ellis J, *et al*. Comparison of efficacy of ciprofloxacin and doxycycline against experimental melioidosis and glanders. *J Antimicrob Chemother* 2000; 45: 813–818.

38. Anonymous. Outbreak of acute febrile illness among participants in Eco-Challenge Sabah 2000 – Malaysia, 2000. *MMWR* 2000; 49: 816–817.

39. Seghal S, Sugunan A, Murhekar M, *et al*. Randomized controlled trial of doxycycline prophylaxis against leptospirosis in an endemic area. *Int J Antimicrob Agents* 2000; 13: 249–255.

40. Hollander J E, Singer A J. Laceration management. *Ann Emerg Med* 1999; 34: 356–367.

41. Kumar S, Malecki J M. A case of neonatal tetanus. *South Med J* 1991; 84: 396–398.

42. Panning C A, Bayat M. Generalized tetanus in a patient with a diabetic foot infection. *Pharmacotherapy* 1999; 19: 885–890.

43. Present D A, Meislin R, Shaffer B. Gas gangrene. A review. *Orthop Rev* 1990; 19: 333–341.

44. Valentine E G. Nontraumatic gas gangrene. *Ann Emerg Med* 1997; 30: 109–111.

45. Korhonen K, Klossner J, Hirn M. Management of clostridial gas gangrene and the role of hyperbaric oxygen. *Ann Chir Gynaecol* 1999; 88: 139–142.

46. BBC News Online. Killer heroin inquiry delayed. http://news.bbc.co.uk (4 June 2001.)

3

Zoonoses of agricultural animals

Despite the well-publicised setbacks that the agricultural sector has experienced in the last few years, there is still a large and active indigenous farming and livestock operation in the British Isles. Eggs, milk and meat are currently produced in quantity for human consumption.

In June 1998, the Ministry of Agriculture, Fisheries, and Food (MAFF: now the Department for Environment, Food, and Rural Affairs (DEFRA)) estimated there were 147.6 million fowl (hens, chickens, pheasants, ducks, etc.), 11.5 million cattle (dairy or beef), 44.5 million sheep and 8.1 million pigs in the UK. This number, although slightly altered by events since, represents a fairly accurate estimate of the numbers today (Table 3.1). Table 3.2 shows the number of animals slaughtered during the recent foot-and-mouth outbreak.

The Health and Safety Executive, who have responsibility for the safety of agricultural and other workers in this sector, reported in *Farmwise* 2001 that there were more than 20 000 cases annually of people employed in agriculture suffering from zoonotic conditions.

Table 3.1 Provisional figures for number of livestock for each country in the UK, June 1999

	England	Wales	Scotland	N Ireland	UK
Cattle	6 342 210	1 318 340	2 044 280	1 718 540	11 423 360
Sheep	20 273 590	11 768 460	9 705 320	2 908 880	44 656 240
Pig	6 163 440	81 540	548 640	490 270	7 283 900
Poultry[a]	128 667 390	10 588 500	10 938 170	15 047 890	165 241 950
Goats	56 870	7 870	8 860	3 570	77 160
Deer	24 640	800	8 040	2 800	36 280
Horses	206 670	34 230	26 140	9 860	276 890

[a]Includes turkeys, ducks, geese and guinea fowl and also includes ostriches in England and Wales.

These figures predate the outbreak of foot-and-mouth disease that resulted in mass slaughter of cattle, sheep and pigs (see Table 3.2).

Figures courtesy of the Department for Environment, Food, and Rural Affairs (http://www.defra.gov.uk).

Table 3.2 Number of animals slaughtered during the recent foot-and-mouth outbreak in the UK

Animal	Number slaughtered
Sheep	3 199 000
Cattle	598 000
Pigs	147 000
Goats	2000
Deer	1000
Total slaughtered	3 947 000

Data from the Department for Environment, Food, and Rural Affairs (http://www.defra.gov.uk).

Many of these cases have been reported under the Control of Substances Hazardous to Health (COSHH) regulations, as the causative pathogens fall under the terms of reference for those regulations. Much has been done to reduce the risks associated with zoonotic infection whilst caring for domesticated animals or processing animals and their products from farm to table, but much remains to be done. The provision of protective clothing and equipment and adoption of safe working practices and other safeguards not only protect workers but also the public at large.

Many of the diseases in this chapter have a long historic association with animal husbandry, probably dating from the first domestication of wild species. Many of the pathogens are almost household names and certainly maintain a hold on our collective consciousness, sometimes out of proportion to their current significance. Others are less familiar; nevertheless, they may still pose a risk.

One of the recent developments in agricultural enterprise has been the extended range of animal species kept for commercial purposes, as farms have responded to the changing market by diversifying. These changes in the spectrum of species with which those employed in the industry come into close contact can lead to different zoonotic pathogens becoming more important. The last section of this chapter deals with two such diseases.

Birds

Introduction

Birds kept in agriculture now come from very diverse origins and cover a variety of species across the avian genera. It is hard to come to terms with an industry where not only do traditional poultry have a place, but also the ostrich and the Gressingham duck (a cross between traditional domesticated ducks and the mallard).

In recent years, while there has been a diversification within the poultry farm and other bird-based enterprises, the pattern of farming has also changed. Eggs produced by battery hens can still be seen on supermarket shelves, but in response to consumer pressure the free-range hen and its eggs are making a dramatic comeback on the basis of better animal welfare and improved flavour. Chickens and capons are again being reared solely for the table, rather than as a sideline to the industrial broiler unit.

These changes come at a price to healthcare. The implications for food and its consumption are discussed in Chapter 4: the import for zoonotic disease in poultry workers is slightly different. Any of the zoonotic conditions discussed in Chapter 2 which are capable of affecting companion bird species may also strike domesticated fowl. In addition other conditions are seen in bird flocks.

The change in husbandry practice carries with it the exposure of the birds to a wider environment and with it wild bird species. As yet, this has had no adverse effects on commercial flocks in this country. In contrast, in the USA the West Nile virus (WNV) is now known to be established in turkeys and chickens in the now endemic areas of the eastern seaboard, acting as an animal reservoir for the pathogen.

In the past, wild species were excluded from poultry housing by never allowing birds out and by controlling feral pigeons and other birds from gaining access to feed mills and storage. This probably slowed the spread of possible pathogens, be they zoonotic or not. There is a growing realisation that new patterns of operation may require heightened vigilance and monitoring.

Newcastle disease
(Pseudo fowl pest)

Newcastle disease is caused by avian paramyxovirus type 1 (PMV-1). It is a notifiable disease in poultry and routine vaccination prevents major outbreaks, which historically rapidly wiped out whole flocks.

Disease in animals

The clinical course of the disease is brief; birds often have catastrophic diarrhoea, breathing difficulties and copious mucus discharge from nostrils and mouth. The birds may become comatose and die, although in the most virulent form death is so rapid that few other symptoms are seen.

Transmission

Transmission occurs following inhalation of infected material, such as faecal matter, direct contact with infected birds or their carcasses or live vaccine. Contamination of the conjunctiva can also occur via bird and plumage dusts. Fomites contact in intensive housing with high levels of infection can also lead to transmission.

Disease in humans

Individuals employed within the poultry industry are most at risk. Accidental infection during vaccination occurs occasionally. Slaughterhouse operatives and laboratory workers are also considered to be at risk if they are handling infected birds or clinical samples.[1]

The first clinical symptom of infection in humans is usually a painful self-limiting conjunctivitis. On occasions a debilitating low fever of up to 3 weeks' duration with spontaneous rapid recovery has been reported.

Treatment

Treatment is usually symptomatic. It may include antiviral or antibacterial eye preparations to treat either primary or secondary infection. Aciclovir eye ointment has proved effective in early primary infection, with either chloramphenicol or fusidic acid preparations for controlling any secondary pathogens.

Prevention

Prevention strategies involve thorough and comprehensive vaccinations of all poultry to prevent disease. Poultry workers should wear respirators and face masks when working with flocks and in housing. Precautions should be adopted to prevent accidental inhalation of vaccine droplets during air-carried vaccination procedures, and all housing should be thoroughly cleaned when not in use.

Cattle

Introduction

Cattle are kept around the world for the production of meat, milk and cheese, and hides for leather. Before the outbreak of foot-and-mouth disease (FMD) there were roughly 11.5 million animals in the UK. The number of animals that will remain when the 2000–2001 outbreak is over is not predictable, but the significance of cattle for the agricultural and wider economy of this country will remain.

The zoonotic infections that cattle suffer are particularly important, not only because they are emotive (such as bovine spongiform encephalopathy/variant Creutzfeldt–Jakob disease (BSE/vCJD)), but also because of the widespread consumption of cattle products. Concerted efforts have been made over past decades to reduce the risks of particularly important zoonoses, such as brucellosis and bovine tuberculosis, and the success of the measures taken is demonstrated by the current low incidence of these diseases.

The prion diseases are dealt with in Chapter 5. In this section the diseases discussed are those which have either currently or historically been of particular healthcare importance.

Brucellosis
(Mediterranean fever, undulant fever, Malta fever)

Brucellosis was named after Bruce who in 1887 identified the bacterium that caused Malta dog, a disease familiar to many generations of seafarers. He named this pathogen, which he isolated from goat's milk, *Brucella melitensis*. This is only one of the causatives of the group of diseases that are aggregated under the general name of brucellosis. They are caused by various species of *Brucella*, depending on source of infection and the associated animal host. As our knowledge and exploration of the bacterial fauna of other species have become more extensive, there has been the identification of varieties of *Brucella* associated with species as diverse as dolphins, seals and rats. Other species such as hares have been identified as carriers, capable of infecting other animals, particularly pigs, over wide geographic areas.[2]

The species responsible for most human infections are *B. abortus* from cattle, *B. melitensis* from sheep and goats, *B. canis* from dogs and *B. suis* from pigs. The diseases are distributed worldwide and are particularly prevalent in South America, Africa, the Mediterranean, Asia and Eastern Europe, where large flocks of animals are tended, and where eradication programmes are impracticable or unenforceable. The World Health Organization (WHO) has an ongoing programme of eradication by slaughter and vaccination aimed at controlling the disease in countries around the Mediterranean basin. Significant numbers of cases have been seen in Malta and Oman, where the disease has re-emerged after an eradication campaign which was believed to have freed the countries from the disease. The UK declared eradication in 1993 of *B. abortus*, and the use of pasteurisation, vaccination and slaughter inspection has been successful so far in preventing recurrence. *B. melitensis* has never been isolated from animals in the UK and is therefore not considered to pose a threat. Only a small proportion of dairy produce is derived from goats and sheep in the UK and there is a testing and screening programme in place which constantly monitors for this pathogen.[3]

Disease in animals

In animals the main symptoms in all breeds suffering from the four main zoonotic strains previously mentioned are focal necrosis of the placenta, abortion and future infertility. The birth fluids and afterbirth are highly infective, and cattle on contaminated pasture are infected by grazing ingesting infected material. The disease is inapparent before the heifer aborts. Bulls may also be infected and can sexually transmit the pathogen, until ultimately becoming sterile. Cattle may be infected with any of the zoonotic strains, while horses appear to be resistant to all of the known zoonotic strains.

Disease in humans

Disease in humans usually follows the ingestion of unpasteurised milk or milk products contaminated with either *B. abortus* or *B. melitensis*, and is well documented. An alternative route for infection is by contact with contaminated bodily fluids, membranes or aborted young. There is some evidence for aerosol spread by infected droplets or dusts. There have been isolated reports of human-to-human transmission by sexual contact.[4] Human disease presents with lymph node swelling, enlargement of the spleen, fever, testicular swelling, influenza-like symptoms and lethargy, nausea and weight loss. Endocarditis or meningitis may follow, sometimes with fatal results.[5]

There is also a chronic undulant form which was often seen in cowmen and veterinary surgeons. Periodic bouts of high fever and clinical symptoms are interspersed with periods of remission with no clinical signs. This can persist for years or decades. The use of anti-biotics effects a cure in most cases; however, prolonged therapy may be necessary in refractory cases.

A septicaemic form also exists. There is evidence that this is caused by the inhalation of infected aerosols in abattoirs and meat-processing plants where infected animals or their tissues are processed. It is char-acterised by an acute systemic disease with high fever.

Diagnosis

Diagnosis follows blood culture; polymerase chain reaction (PCR) has also been tried. The bacteria are relatively slow-growing and successful culture in laboratories can prove difficult.

Treatment

Treatment relies on the use of antimicrobials, usually in combination to prevent resistance. The *British National Formulary*[6] and the WHO rec-ommend the use of doxycycline plus rifampicin or streptomycin. In the past co-trimoxazole was often used; associated toxicity has led to its replacement by more suitable agents. Therapy is usually prolonged – the WHO recommends 6 weeks as a minimum duration. The *BNF*[6] recom-mends rifampicin 600 mg to 1.2 g daily in 2–4 divided doses with doxy-cycline 100–200 mg/day; the WHO recommendation is similar – rifampicin 600–900 mg/day plus doxycycline 200 mg. In severe cases streptomycin may be used in place of or in addition to the rifampicin. Longer-term therapy may be required in the undulant form of the disease.

Recently the quinolones in combination with rifampicin have been trialled and demonstrated to be as effective. Currently no effective vac-cine for human brucellosis is available.

Prevention

Suitable protective clothing will reduce the risk from occupational exposure. The use of disinfectants, especially chlorinated, iodine- or ammonia-based products, can prevent environmental hazards. The main-stay of prevention is eradication by animal vaccination or slaughter programmes. On a personal basis, travellers to areas where the disease is endemic should be encouraged to avoid unpasteurised dairy products and undercooked meat.

Foot-and-mouth disease

It is questionable whether FMD is an important zoonosis, although in economic terms for livestock farmers there is absolutely no question of its impact.[7] It does have a zoonotic potential, as a single case in the 1967 outbreak and one confirmed case in the current (2000–2001) outbreak have shown; however, the circumstances leading to human infection are usually extreme.[8]

The disease is found worldwide and all cloven-hoofed animals are affected. Caused by an aphthovirus, there are several different serotypes, of which the most virulent is serotype O (Pan-Asiatic), which is responsible for the current epidemic.

Disease in animals

The first symptom of infection in animals is a high fever; blisters and ulceration develop on the mouth and the feet, leading to lameness and poor feeding ability. The disease spreads rapidly within herds, as infected animals are actively infectious and large amounts of live virus are produced before and after clinical symptoms commence. Piglets are the worst affected, and the disease can cause high mortality.

Spread to other sites is believed to occur on the wind, by physical means, including vehicular, livestock or human movement.

Disease in humans

The WHO has only recorded about 40 confirmed cases of FMD in humans worldwide in the 20th century, of which most have been related to the O serotype. Transmission has been documented following deliberate ingestion of unpasteurised milk from infected cows by three German veterinary surgeons in 1834. In brief, very close contact with infected cattle or their products seems to be necessary for infection to occur.

Following an incubation period of between 2 and 6 days, clinical signs of infection commence. Blisters appear on the hands and sometimes on the feet and in the mouth and/or the tongue. Symptoms normally resolve spontaneously, usually within a week of the last appearance of blistering.[9]

Diagnosis

Confirmation of the diagnosis is made by serology testing on clinical samples.

Treatment

There is no treatment except symptomatic support. Prevention of disease in humans is normally managed by protective clothing for personnel handling or culling infected animals, and the pasteurisation of dairy products. A vaccine is available for animal use; however, there are a variety of issues surrounding herd vaccination programmes which need careful consideration. Vaccinated cattle may not be exported to countries where FMD is not endemic and the ability of a country to gain or regain 'disease-free' status may be compromised by the routine use of vaccination.

Prevention

Prevention of FMD in animals relies upon a host of organisations. Importation of infected foodstuffs, which then entered the animal food chain following inadequate heat treatment of swill, was probably the source of the latest outbreak. HM Customs and Excise are tasked with controlling this trade, but individual travellers may illegally import meat or meat products or contaminated dairy products into the UK in their luggage, making the task of control well-nigh impossible. Importation of contaminated livestock has also been suggested as a means of spread, and outbreaks in continental Europe have been linked to infected livestock exported from the UK.

Locally, disinfectant in foot and vehicular baths helps prevent physical transfer. DEFRA provides a list of disinfectants which are approved under the Diseases of Animals (Approved Disinfectants) 1978 as amended for use against FMD and/or in respect of General Orders (25 April 2001).

Once an outbreak occurs and is notified to DEFRA (previously MAFF) it becomes the lead organisation, and is responsible for all aspects of disease control. The discussion between this department and other representative organisations of farmers and the livestock industry around vaccination and/or culling is still raging fiercely at the time of publication, and will continue for the foreseeable future.

Other issues

Media misconceptions have much to do with the publicity this condition has received. There is another virus of the coxsackie family that produces similar symptoms in children called hand, foot and mouth disease, which leads to confusion, as may infection with other viral pathogens.

In Chapter 1, the impact of other aspects of zoonotic disease on human populations was discussed. FMD has profound implications for people employed in agriculture and the food industry. Bankruptcy, redundancy or short-time working, with associated loss of livelihood, housing and work, are all factors likely to lead to mental health problems requiring healthcare support. The farming community has suffered much in recent years, especially in the livestock trade, and suicides have become more frequent.[8]

The disposal of carcasses may also pose a public health hazard. Due to the scale of this last outbreak, there have been incidents of considerable time elapsing between slaughter and burial or burning of animal corpses. The decomposition of animals and the associated human distress pose a health risk not only in terms of the immediate environment, but also for affected individuals who may suffer long-term mental health problems.[9]

Disposal of carcasses by burning leads to hazards associated with the smoke, smell, particulate contamination and high atmospheric levels of combustion products, including dioxins, being produced. The impact on the local population of the sights and scenes of disposal can lead to distress. This is also true for personnel involved in the screening, slaughtering and disposal process.

Case histories

The two confirmed human cases in the UK – the first in the 1966 outbreak and the other in 2001 – bear examination, if only to emphasise how difficult it is to catch the disease.

In 1966, a 35-year-old agricultural machinery salesman, Bobby Brewis, lived on a farm at Yetlington, Northumberland, with his brother. The cattle on the farm were slaughtered, having developed FMD. Mr Brewis took no part in the slaughter, but watched from some distance. Later he developed the symptoms of the disease. On being diagnosed he fainted, believing he would be shot, like the infected cattle. It is unclear how he became infected, but it is believed he may have consumed milk derived from the infected herd.

As a result he was ostracised by the local community, lost his job and was last heard of as a fish-and-chip shop proprietor in Sunderland.

Details of the 2001 case are sketchier, with a confirmed case in a contract worker employed to cull cattle in Cumbria. From the details released, it would appear that the man was contaminated whilst dealing with a carcass. Material from the dead or dying animal sprayed the man copiously, and he later developed symptoms of the disease. As a spokesman for the Public Health Laboratory Service (PHLS) so neatly put it, 'if you place a human being in contact with that size of inoculum, there is always a chance they will develop the disease'.

Q fever
(Query fever, Balkan influenza, abattoir fever)

Q fever, first described in Australia in the 1950s, is a disease that stems from cattle, although it usually causes no symptoms in the host animal. It is caused by a rickettsia, *Coxiella burnetii*, an obligate intracellular bacterium. The causative organism has a global distribution and it is possible for many species, including ticks, fleas and lice, as well as many vertebrates, to carry the disease. The main significant zoonotic reservoir is considered to be bovines and also sheep. Once infected the organism colonises and produces infective foci in the mammary glands and the placenta of pregnant animals. During birth large quantities of the organism can be found in the amniotic fluid and on the placenta. The organism is capable of forming an environmentally resistant spore form capable of forming the inoculum for delayed outbreaks. Surveys carried out on dairy herds in England and Wales suggest that up to 20% of all stock may be infected.[10]

The presence of the organism in milk results from the colonisation of the mammary system, and host animals can carry the disease for prolonged periods, with shedding occurring sporadically or constantly during lactation. The organism is resistant to heat and ideal pasteurisation conditions will remove it from milk; however, there is a risk from unpasteurised or incompletely pasteurised milk or milk products. It has been postulated that urine and faeces from infected animals may also be a carrier medium for the organism.

Sixty-four cases of Q fever were reported in England during 1998, and 44 in Northern Ireland. Interestingly, most cases in Northern Ireland were in male agricultural workers who were probably exposed to the pathogen in the course of their work.

Transmission

Transmission to humans usually follows exposure to infected material and DEFRA considers it to be an occupational zoonosis of agricultural and other workers closely involved with cattle and sheep. The people at highest risk are veterinary surgeons and stock people who assist at births, although the organism is highly resistant to desiccation and therefore can infect individuals working with hides, fleece or the bones of infected animals. Transmission is by direct contact with contaminated materials, especially the afterbirth or material contaminated with amniotic fluid. There is some evidence that inhalation of dust from infected straw or bedding and even soil may also cause infection. Further down the food-processing chain, transport drivers and abattoir workers may also be at risk. Drinking milk or consuming contaminated milk products is also a possible route of infection, and transmission via ticks, lice or fleas has been demonstrated.[11]

Disease in humans

Most exposed individuals display no signs of clinical disease. Infection rates and recording of clinical cases correspond to lambing and calving cycles, allowing for the time lag associated with the organism's incubation period. After infection there is an incubation period of between 2 and 4 weeks followed by an acute onset with high fever, associated chills, profuse sweating and severe headache. Unlike other rickettsial diseases, in humans there is no skin rash. The patient may also present with anorexia, sickness and lethargy. The fever may last anything from 9 to 14 days and can recur at intervals, with a total duration of up to 3 months. A dry cough may also be present, with pain in the chest cavity similar to pleuritic pain. 'Cracking' in the chest may also be heard during respiration. Lesions in the lungs may be apparent on X-ray examination. Liver enlargement or tenderness with associated hepatitis-type symptoms can be seen.

Untreated cases can resolve within 5–14 days, although symptoms may not regress for more than 7–8 weeks and relapses may occur. The untreated fatality rate is estimated at 1% of cases. Following severe infection there may be a need for prolonged convalescence. Elderly patients are particularly badly affected by this disease and may require prolonged supportive measures.

A chronic form also exists which causes a prolonged endocarditis leading to valvular damage, especially of the aortic valve. Recent figures show that damage is more common in patients with pre-existing valve damage. Symptoms can appear long after the disease has run its clinical course and may require replacement of damaged valves. The fatality associated with this form is estimated to be as high as 60% of cases unless corrective surgery is undertaken. Chronic hepatitis also develops in a small number of cases.

Diagnosis

Diagnosis follows serological testing, as the organism is slow-growing and almost impossible to culture from clinical specimens.

Treatment

C. burnetii can be difficult to treat as it can show a lack of response, rather than true resistance to antibiotics. The *BNF*[6] recommends the use of tetracyclines at usual clinical dose, and historically chloramphenicol has been used, although it is reserved for recalcitrant infections due to the incidence of major side-effects. The length of the course may require adjustment so that therapy is extended for a period of days after the fever regresses to prevent relapse. Patients with endocarditis and valvular damage will need prolonged prophylaxis up to and beyond surgery, with valve replacement or repair. Studies have shown that the organism has a heightened susceptibility to combinations of drugs which result in acidification of the intracellular vacuole. Chloroquine in combination with doxycycline has been used with some notable success.

Prevention

As with many other zoonoses, prevention strategies revolve around good personal and environmental hygiene. Bedding contaminated by postpartum material and the material itself should be carefully handled, with collection and subsequent burying or incineration. Disinfection of housing and other areas should be carried out with DEFRA-approved products. Protective clothing, including respirators, overalls and gloves, must be worn wherever feasible. In the USA a vaccine for cattle has been developed; it is not licensed for use in the UK. Carrier animals have been subject to eradication by slaughter policy. Nevertheless, the organism is considered to be widespread in the environment and preventing animals from becoming infected is deemed to be practically impossible. All milk and milk products should be pasteurised, and monitoring of the process should be maintained in the normal manner to ensure that optimal temperatures and duration standards are met.

Tapeworm

The beef tapeworm (*Taenia saginata*, also known as *Cysticercus bovis*) and the pork tapeworm *(T. solium)* are very similar both in overall appearance and life cycle. They are both members of the cestode worm family. The definitive host for both worms is humans: the tapeworm only reaches maturity in the lumen of the human gut. The associated animal is an intermediate host which is necessary for the larvae to infect humans after ingesting infected inadequately cooked meat from a suspect carcass. Comparison with *Echinococcus granulosus* may be of interest (see pp. 57–59). It is also a cestode, but in this case humans are blind intermediate hosts, and the usual cycle uses dogs as a primary host and sheep as a full intermediate host – the exact reverse of *Taenia*.[12]

In 1998 there were 59 reports received at the Communicable Disease Surveillance Centre (CSDC) of human infection with *Taenia* spp. Of these, 37 were confirmed as *T. saginata*, and the rest were not speciated. Of the patients, 17 were travellers and were considered to have become infected whilst abroad. There have been no reported cases of *T. solium* in the UK since 1994.

General parasitology

The adult worm is flat in cross-section and widens gradually from the head or scolex, through the proglottids or body segments. The scolex attaches to the gut wall of the host by means of suckers and/or hooks, depending on the species involved (Plate 4).

The body segments or proglottids are produced from just behind the scolex, and the oldest and most mature are at the opposite end of the worm. As the segments mature they develop both male and female reproductive organs, self-fertilise and produce eggs which are contained within the proglottid wall. The mature proglottids break away from the body (or strobila, consisting of all the proglottids and the scolex) and pass out of the gut via the anus. The secondary or intermediate host, in which the larvae can develop, is then infected by ingestion of either the eggs or embryos present in faecal matter.

The tapeworm absorbs nutrients from the gut of the host over its whole body surface, and has a rudimentary nervous and digestive system. The worms are host-specific and exist as an adult solely in the gut of their preferred host. When eggs hatch in the gut of a host, either primary or intermediate, larvae penetrate the wall of the gut, and then migrate to a preferred site, usually in muscle tissue or other organs. In either pigs or cattle these normally migrate and encyst again in muscle tissue, where the cyst may develop daughter cysts with multiple internal scolices.

Alternatively they may migrate to other organs and cause a condition known as cysticercosis. The larvae encyst in sites as diverse as the brain or other areas of the central nervous system, eyelid and conjunctiva. The condition is seen mainly in intermediate hosts, but may also be seen in humans, where either eggs or larvae are ingested, or where the gravid proglottid (a mature proglottid full of eggs or embryos) ruptures in the gut before it can be expelled.

In cysticercosis, the cysts may be quiescent or active. Where active cysts are present they undergo a budding and proliferation process, called racemose cysticercosis, leading to a series of connected cysts with multiple scolices in the vacuole. When the cysts are sited in the brain complications, including neurological disturbances with epilepsy or paraesthesia, can occur. Hydrocephalus may also be present if cysts occlude structures in the brain.

Disease in humans

Adult beef worms can reach a size of between 12.5 and 25 metres in length; the pork tapeworm is much smaller, only reaching between 2 and 7 metres. They are usually solitary occupants of any infested gut as multiple worms can cause intestinal obstruction. The beef tapeworm differs from the pork tapeworm in having no hooks on the scolex. Both species are capable of producing a strobila of 1000–2000 proglottids, and can live for up to 25 years. There are few symptoms associated with the adult worm, except slight irritation of the site of attachment or vague abdominal symptoms with hunger pangs, loss of weight and general condition, indigestion, diarrhoea and/or constipation. Discomfort and embarrassment may be caused by migrating proglottids when they reach the anus. The proglottids may be seen with the naked eye, either grouped or as single segments in the stool. The proglottids may be mobile when moist, becoming quiescent as they become desiccated.

The beef tapeworm rarely causes cysticercosis; however the pork tapeworm can cause this condition in humans. Definite diagnosis of infestation either follows isolation of eggs or proglottids from the stool or protrusion of a portion of the strobila through the anal sphincter.

Serological testing using enzyme-linked immunosorbent assay (ELISA) methods confirms diagnosis, and in cases of cysticercosis, imaging by computed tomography, radiology or magnetic resonance is usually necessary. Biopsy of subcutaneous cysticerci will also confirm other findings.

The symptoms of neurocysticercosis depend upon the number of lesions present and their location, size and status. Live foci are usually asymptomatic: as the cysts degenerate and die there is a progressive inflammatory response causing encephalitis and swelling. Epileptic seizures are the most frequent symptom. Meningitis, raised intracranial pressure and paraesthesia may also occur.

Treatment

For adult tapeworms treatment is undertaken using either niclosamide or praziquantel. The *BNF*[6] states that niclosamide is available from IDIS Ltd on a named-patient basis. It is solely active against adult worms and does not kill larval stages. Side-effects are usually limited to gastro-intestinal disturbances and itching with occasional rash. To prevent any risk of cysticercosis by autoinfection following emesis, an antiemetic should be given at the same time as the niclosamide, on wakening.

Praziquantel is available from Merck on a named-patient basis. It is deemed to be as effective as niclosamide, and should be given at a single dose of 10–20 mg/kg of body weight after a light breakfast.

There is some controversy surrounding treatment of cysticercosis. Usually surgical removal of the cysts is advocated in humans before damage ensues, with concomitant administration of anthelmintics. This is very important in infection associated with the eyes.[13]

In central nervous system involvement, symptom control of associated epilepsy is achieved using the usual anticonvulsants. The *BNF*[6] does not make any recommendations on the use of anthelmintics (or cestocides) in neurocysticercosis; however, elsewhere in the world praziquantel or albendazole has been routinely used. Albendazole is a benzimidazole anthelmintic and is approved for treatment of only hydatid disease and neurocysticercosis in the USA. It is teratogenic in animals, so a careful risk/benefit analysis must be carried out before it is used in women who are pregnant or of child-bearing years. It is hepatotoxic, and can also destroy bone marrow, therefore complete blood chemistry analyses and liver function tests should be routinely carried out before and during therapy.[14]

To obtain a cestocidal effect praziquantel at a dose of 50 mg/kg per day three times daily by mouth for 2 weeks or albendazole at 15 mg/kg orally two to three times a day for 8–15 days depending on radiological findings has been shown to destroy viable cysts. Symptomatic treatment is also necessary to ensure good clinical outcome.

Because of the nature of the condition, clinical trials have proved problematic and a recent Cochrane Review[14] has been unable to find evidence of dramatic advantages in using anthelmintic treatment and supportive therapy over purely supportive therapy in terms of clinical outcome. The measures used included the incidence of hydrocephalus, reduction in use of anticonvulsants and levels of disability or death in cohorts of patients.

Treatment may cause inflammatory changes around foci, which may cause temporary clinical deterioration of the patient, and occasionally where heavy infection is present, death may ensue. Corticosteroids are routinely used as an adjunct to therapy to reduce this inflammatory response. There is therefore an unresolved debate concerning the utility of anthelmintic therapy, especially as there may be severe adverse reactions to the drugs.

Prevention

Tapeworm infection is not common in the UK, due to a strict system of meat inspection. This is not true of the rest of western Europe. Germany and France report significant numbers of cases annually associated with the consumption of infected meat in national delicacies. In non-Muslim developing countries there is a high incidence of the disease, causing more than a third of all cases of adult-onset epilepsy. Due to the longevity of the parasite, immigrants from these countries could present with symptoms of the disease long after their arrival in the UK. In the USA there have been sufficient cases among migrant workers for the condition of cysticercosis to be routinely tested in cases of epilepsy amongst this sociological group. The numbers of tourists travelling from the UK to areas of risk, such as South-east Asia, the Indian subcontinent and Africa, have increased dramatically in the past decade, therefore tapeworm infestation should be excluded in any diagnostic path relating to persistent abdominal symptoms or seizures following such trips.

Suspect meat or meat products should be thoroughly cooked, avoiding wherever possible eating meat which is either raw or undercooked from dubious sources. Suspect carcasses or meat should be frozen for at least 3 weeks to kill any larvae. Viable eggs or embryos may also be present in water contaminated by faecal matter; the usual precautions when drinking water of unknown quality should be applied.

Separation of human sewage and intermediate host animals is important in breaking the infective cycle. Sewage sludge should not be used to dress pasture where animals destined for human consumption are actively grazing or housed. Care should be taken after flooding where there is a possible risk of human sewage contaminating pasture.

Bovine tuberculosis

Although the prime cause of tuberculosis in humans is *Mycobacterium tuberculosis* (var. *hominis*), there are still some cases recorded annually of the condition being caused by the closely related organism M. *bovis*. Clinical signs and symptoms seen in the infection are identical regardless of which of the two mycobacteria are present. The disease can also infect a large number of other mammal species, and has become a source of bitterly contested debate between cattle farmers and wildlife groups in the UK over the role of badgers as a reservoir of infection.

Disease in animals

The primary reservoir of M. *bovis* was historically cattle. Early control measures were focused on improving herd hygiene, culling infected beasts and preventing spread within herds. The most effective control measure was the development of reliable pasteurisation of milk, the primary source of transfer of infection from cattle to humans.

Within cattle herds the disease is transferred by aerosol inhalation with subsequent pulmonary infection, in addition, infection from cow to calf has been well documented, as has reinfection of tuberculosis-free herds by infected humans. Badgers suffering from the disease have long been suspected of infecting cattle. The hard scientific evidence is sketchy, and the mechanism of transmission is as yet unproven. The bacterium has also been found in many other species of animal, both in the UK and elsewhere in the world, with pigs, sheep, goats, horses, cats, dogs and foxes all being capable of carrying infection in endemic areas.

Cattle have been compulsorily and routinely tested using the tuberculin skin test since the 1950s. Beasts with a positive test are slaughtered mandatorily under the Tuberculosis Orders (1984) made under the Animal Health Act 1981. The provision within the legislation for agreed valuation and compensation payments to farmers has been a major asset in achieving farmers' agreement to the measures. Investigation of herds may also stem from veterinary slaughterhouse inspection of cattle and carcasses.

Testing frequency depends upon known regional prevalence, and has led to the UK achieving disease-free status. Devon, Cornwall, the West Midlands, South Wales and Northern Ireland have the highest current incidence of the disease in cattle; the level has risen since an all-time low in the 1980s. In 1998, of approximately 69 000 herds of cattle tested across the whole of the UK, there were just over 1800 individual confirmed cases within the herds. It should be understood that the disease is only controlled, not eradicated.

Clinical signs in cattle are variable. Some animals rapidly lose condition and cough, and there may be udder involvement in dairy cattle. Other cattle may remain sleek and healthy; it was not unknown in the past for the best-looking beast in a herd to be the most infective. Ulcers may be seen in a cutaneous form of the disease that can affect some animals, usually with advanced disease. Generalised symptoms may be seen, with diarrhoea and enlargement of the liver and spleen. Pulmonary disease normally develops from a soft cough to haemoptysis. Physical examination of the walls of stalls for blood-stained mucus was a very primitive method of determining infection in animals, and fortunately this has now been superseded. Any of the other major organs can become affected, and persistent, extensive lymph node swelling may be present. Skeletal involvement can also occur. Paralysis of the hindquarters may occur in some cases.

Transmission

Transmission normally follows the ingestion of inadequately or non-pasteurised infected milk or dairy produce. Stock handlers are also at significantly elevated risk if their charges are infected. Transmission may follow inhalation of infected aerosols, or skin contact with cutaneous lesions on infected animals. In the UK only 25 cases of confirmed human infection were reported in 1998; in two of the cases multiple-drug-resistant *M. bovis* was responsible. There was nothing to link any of the cases with diseased cattle, so these may represent reactivated disease contracted at an earlier date.

Elsewhere in the world control programmes have not been as effective in cattle, so there is a risk of infection following ingestion of dairy produce, especially in developing countries.

Disease in humans

Clinical symptoms vary depending on the source of contamination or route of infection, although this is not always associated. General symptoms include weight loss, pronounced fatigue and fever, all of which may gradually worsen. The classic pulmonary pattern of the disease may be seen with cough and haemoptysis. Ulcers or other lesions may be present in cutaneous disease. As with cattle, the organism can colonise any or all of the major organs or the skeleton, producing symptoms related to site and severity of infected foci.

Patients may be asymptomatic for long periods after infection. Activation and progression of disease may then occur when disease or age affects the immune system. Many of the current cases are among elderly people who were infected in their youth. The disease poses a considerable risk, along with other mycobacterial infection, to patients suffering from human immunodeficiency virus (HIV)/acquired immunodeficiency syndrome (AIDS). Other people at an enhanced risk of contracting the disease are veterinary and animal workers. Migrant workers and members of other immigrant groups may also have the disease; however, as treatment of *M. bovis* and *M. tuberculosis* is the same, drug therapy of one will normally eradicate the other.[15]

Diagnosis

Diagnosis follows positive skin reaction to tuberculin purified protein derivative (PPD). Bacille Calmette-Guérin (BCG) inoculation produces a positive test, so this must be excluded. Radiographic imaging, sputum testing or ELISA assay of samples supports the findings from skin testing. Differentiation of the causative *Mycobacterium* usually follows growth of the organism; however, this can be difficult. Polymerase chain reaction assay has been used to this end, with considerable success.

Treatment

The treatment of infection with *M. bovis* is identical to that for *M. tuberculosis*, and should be carried out by specialist centres. The regimens suggested by the Joint Tuberculosis Committee of the British Thoracic Society are normally used in the UK, and are regularly updated as data relating to prevalence of resistant serotypes is forthcoming. It is not appropriate for the regimens to be discussed in detail as these change rapidly, so the reader is referred to the latest edition of the *BNF* for recommendations.

Prevention

Prevention in animals revolves around the cattle scheme, as outlined above. Other animals may contract the disease and are usually destroyed if found to be positive for the disease.

Personnel at particular risk should wear protective clothing when handling suspect animals, and must be immunised whenever possible.

Bacille Calmette-Guérin (BCG) vaccine is made from a live attenuated strain of *M. bovis,* and is routinely used to immunise people against contracting tuberculosis from both animal and human sources. Most people will have received the immunisation as a teenager. If they have not, they should receive it, especially if they are in a high-risk category, with one notable exception. The vaccine has been reported as causing cases of clinical disease in HIV-positive patients. Therefore such patients should not receive this immunisation. HIV-positive patients who travel to countries where *M. bovis* is endemic should be advised to boil all milk and abstain from any dairy produce that has not been pasteurised or cooked.[16]

Sheep

Introduction

Historically, the UK has always been a prolific producer of wool. In the 17th century, sheep were known as 'God's own animal', not only because of associated Christian symbolism but also as the sheep gave wool for textiles, meat for the table and milk or cheese. There are many varieties of sheep, and many have been specially bred for fleece or meat quality. Other breeds have been developed for hardiness in large areas of the UK, especially in upland areas in the North or in Wales where no other agricultural enterprise is possible due to the poor quality of the land and its pasture.

There were approximately 44 500 000 sheep in the whole of the UK in June 1999, before the foot-and-mouth epidemic. The number has been considerably reduced by the mass slaughter programme; however there is still a significant number of sheep in the fields and on the hills.

Because of the numbers of animals involved, and the amount of human contact sheep receive, especially when lambing, there are a number of zoonotic conditions that are particularly important. It will come as no surprise that most cases of these diseases are reported from rural areas, and knowledge of these conditions is especially important in these regions.

Chlamydiosis
(Gestational psittacosis)

Infection with *Chlamydia psittaci* has already been discussed in Chapter 2. Chlamydiae are all intracellular dwelling parasites and have a strange biphasic reproductive cycle, in which only one phase is infective. It is unclear whether the *Chlamydia* responsible for infection in sheep and goats is a strain of *C. psittaci*, or a separate species *C. pecorum*, as the serological and PCR tests used for diagnosis are not sensitive enough to produce species differentiation.

Disease in animals

The strain found in sheep, goats and occasionally cattle causes a chronic infection, particularly in female animals. The disease in sheep is known as enzootic abortion, and in flocks with high incidence of infection is a major cause of economic losses due to low numbers of live-birthed lambs. It is usually isolated from the uterus and reproductive organs. In pregnant animals it causes placental insufficiency and abortion. The infection appears to be transmitted between animals by either the sexual or the faecal–oral route. Infected animals pass live organism in the faeces, and after abortion or birth the organism is found plentifully in the uterus, vagina and placental material. Lambs may also be contaminated, especially whilst still wet and before maternal cleaning has occurred. The incidence rate in sheep is not known; however, in 1998, out of 2984 diagnoses of sheep abortion in the UK, this organism was implicated in 1082 ewes. Numbers of cases of abortion in sheep related to *C. psittaci* in the last decade have ranged between 1000 and 1700 annually.

Transmission

Transmission to humans follows inhalation of dried faecal matter, direct contact with faeces or contact with pregnant or postpartum ewes,

lambs, birth fluids or placental tissue. The organism is capable of surviving desiccation and survives in dung or soil for several months.

Disease in humans

Following infection there is normally a 1–2-week prepatent period. The
disease usually then presents as an influenza-like illness with cough and
congestion followed by high fever, aching muscles and occasional back
and abdominal pain. Respiratory symptoms are common, with dry
cough and pneumonia. Anaemia and liver dysfunction with hepatic and
splenic enlargement may also be present.

In pregnant women the disease may be life-threatening. This form
was first identified and reported in the UK in 1967, and is luckily rare.
The disease can progress to give placental insufficiency, neonatal distress
and late term miscarriage or premature birth. In some cases, emergency
termination may be necessary to save the mother's life. Disseminated
clotting may occur in all major blood vessels.[17,18]

Diagnosis

Diagnosis is usually made using immunofluorescence techniques, ELISA
or PCR tests.

Treatment

Tetracyclines or erythromycin are the drugs of choice. Erythromycin is
preferable in pregnant women as tetracyclines are contraindicated in
pregnancy, although in resistant cases they may need to be used where
the benefits of treatment outweigh the risks. Caesarean section at early
term may also be necessary.

Prevention

Sheep may be vaccinated to reduce the incidence of enzootic abortion
and shedding of organisms. Suitable protective clothing should be worn,
including face protection, when handling pregnant ewes. Ewes that have
aborted should be isolated until any vaginal discharge ceases.

Pregnant women should, wherever possible, avoid contact with
pre-, peri- or postpartum ewes or goats, and kids or lambs. Contact
with placental material or aborted lambs must be avoided. They should

not handle unwashed overalls that may be contaminated with blood or secretions from ewes or lambs, or milk ewes. Any pregnant woman who has been in contact with sheep should seek medical advice if she has an onset of influenza-like symptoms or fever.

Additional notes

There is another strain of *C. psittaci*, feline keratoconjunctivitis agent, which typically causes rhinitis, pneumonia or conjunctivitis in cats. This strain can also be transmitted to humans, but it is extremely rare. The resulting conjunctivitis responds to the use of antibiotic eyedrops or eye ointment, particularly chlortetracycline or fusidic acid.

Giardiasis

Giardiasis is caused by the flagellate protozoan *Giardia lamblia*. It has a worldwide distribution and, although humans are one of the main reservoir for the disease, it is considered to be zoonotic as sheep, cattle, pigs, dogs, birds such as budgerigars and parrots and other species are also known to harbour the parasite. It is a biphasic protozoan having an encysted and a free-living or trophozite form. The trophozite is killed by gastric acid so only the encysted form poses a risk of infection to humans. The disease is endemic in developing countries where it is prevalent in most animals and children. Giardiasis is recognised not only as an issue for public health, but also as a traveller's zoonosis and as an infection of other risk groups domestically.[19]

Disease in animals

Infected animals may be asymptomatic; alternatively they may have weight loss with chronic diarrhoea and partially formed fatty stools. The parasite matures and reproduces in the host's intestine and is then passed with the stool. Once expelled the cysts can survive adverse environmental conditions for prolonged periods.

Transmission

Faecal contamination of water or food and its subsequent consumption by humans is the most common route of infection. Water from wells or other ground systems can be contaminated with faecal matter, and when either unfiltered or inadequately filtered before consumption poses a significant risk. Tap water in countries with poor infrastructure support can also be a source of infection.[20]

The oral–faecal route of infection is also common, especially in children. The cysts are infectious virtually immediately they are passed in the stool so person-to-person spread can occur as a result of poor personal hygiene. This can be of particular importance in care settings, such as day care, nurseries and other premises. Fomites spread by faecal contamination of surfaces or objects is well documented.

In addition to young children and elderly people living in communal settings, the other risk groups are travellers (especially those on a budget using poor-quality accommodation or eating in substandard venues), outdoor enthusiasts, sexually active male homosexuals and the immunocompromised. Patients with HIV will often present with giardial infection; it is not clear if this significantly affects clinical outcomes or survival times.[21]

Disease in humans

The inoculum necessary to produce clinical disease has been estimated at as low as a single viable cyst, making it extremely infective. Following ingestion the cysts hatch in the small intestine. They can live free in the gut lumen or can attach to the gut wall. The parasite reproduces rapidly and encysts as it progresses towards the large intestine. Infection may be asymptomatic; in other patients clinical signs appear after a prepatent period of between 1 and 4 weeks.

The disease may present as diarrhoea of either chronic or acute nature, of either mild or severe character. Unlike other organisms, the stools are associated with considerable gas and are usually fatty, frothy and evil-smelling. They are usually free from blood or mucus. There is associated bloating, gastrointestinal spasm and abdominal pain. The patient may feel weary, nauseous, and report loss of weight and appetite. Dehydration may occur.

Untreated, the condition normally lasts for 1–2 weeks. Some individuals can develop a chronic form of the disease which may last for months or years, which leads to chronic malabsorption states with associated anorexia. Disaccharide intolerance may develop in nearly 40% of any giardial sufferers during and for up to 6 months following infection. Once resolved, infection seems to confer some immunity against reinfection.

Diagnosis

Diagnosis has traditionally been by isolating viable cysts from faecal material of suspected sufferers. An ELISA test is now available, as is a fluorescent antibody test, which simplifies rapid confirmation of clinical findings.

Treatment

Metronidazole is the treatment of choice for giardiasis – either 2 g/day for 3 days or 400 mg three times a day for 5 days. Alternatively, tinidazole as a single dose of 2 g or mepacrine hydrochloride 100 mg every 8 hours for 5–7 days can be used. Mepacrine is unlicensed in the UK for this condition; however, it is available on a named-patient basis or as a special item from BCM (address below). As previously mentioned, rehydration therapy may be necessary as an adjunct to other therapy.

Chronic cases are often refractory, requiring repeated treatment courses to achieve elimination of the protozoan.

Prevention

The following general advice is applicable to many faecal-borne pathogens, and also forms a backbone of good practice for travellers. In countries where the disease is endemic or suspected, only drink bottled water and avoid drinking water or consuming foods which have not been washed in bottled water. Hot drinks, prepacked carbonated drinks and pasteurised items are usually safe. Ice in drinks made from local water should be avoided. Only fruit or vegetables which have a peel or can be peeled and then washed should be consumed. Any vegetables should be washed in bottled or boiled water and adequately cooked.

When consuming water from a suspect source is the only alternative, water purification tablets should be used or the water should be boiled before consumption.

Domestically, normal hygiene routines of washing hands after defecating and before handling food prevent spread. For care workers and others working where faecal contamination of patients or objects is commonplace, wearing gloves and ensuring personal hygiene is observed aid prevention of infection and also spread.

Individuals with HIV should be encouraged to have their companion animals tested for giardiasis regularly and treated to eliminate the organism if present. Objects, areas and materials contaminated with animal faeces should be disinfected and cleaned. In severely immuno-compromised individuals, pets may need to be housed permanently indoors to prevent reinfection.

Useful address

BCM Specials Manufacturing
D10 First 114
Nottingham NG20 2PR
Tel: +44 (0) 800 952 1010

Orf
(Contagious pustular dermatitis)

Orf is caused by a parapoxvirus of the Poxviridae family. It is endemic in sheep and goats and occurs globally; some herds are completely free of the organism. At present there is considerable discussion as to whether the incidence of the disease has been increased by the vaccination of herds where there was previously no history of cases.

Disease in animals

In sheep or goats, crusty lesions on or around the muzzle, eyelids, mouth, feet or external genitalia may be laden with virus. Necrosis of the skin of the gastrointestinal and urogenital tract can occur. The virus is shed by infected animals in secretions from lesions and also in faeces and urine. The virus is persistent in the environment and may survive for many years.

Transmission

Orf is an uncommon disease in humans; however, it is easily transmitted by contact with lesions on animals or infected wool. Accidental infection with live vaccine during vaccination of sheep also poses a risk.

Disease in humans

Following infection, ulcerative suppurating lesions on face, hands and arms appear. Shepherds, sheep shearers and others who handle live sheep, warm carcasses or unprocessed fleeces or wool are at risk. During

1998, 60 incidents relating to accidental vaccination in humans were reported.[22]

Treatment

Treatment is purely supportive, as there is no therapy recommended. Lesions usually regress within 6–8 weeks with minimal scarring. Secondary infection of sores may occur and management using antiseptics or antibiotics may be required.

Prevention

Good hygiene practices and wearing rubber gloves when handling infected sheep helps to prevent infection in individuals at risk due to their occupation. Fomites contact may also be responsible for spread, and prevention strategies centre around good disinfection procedures. Care when using the live attenuated vaccine to vaccinate flocks is essential.[23]

Pigs

Introduction

Although the domestic pig industry has gone through a difficult period in the last decade, there are still approximately 7 250 000 pigs in the UK, of which over 6 million are in England. Much of the industry still focuses on the intensive pig unit, using selectively bred animals geared to the requirements of producers for rapid growth and consumers for lean bacon and pork.

With the reduction in grain prices, and the programme of set-aside land, more acreage in the UK has become available for outside pig enterprises. This has the added advantage for producers that they are able to gain higher returns on their products as it satisfies the demands for high welfare products by consumer lobby groups. It has also enabled producers to return to using older breeds of pig, with a reduction in the therapeutic interventions and medicated foodstuffs associated with intensive enterprise.

It should also not be forgotten that some producers have switched to wild boar or boar/pig hybrids in an attempt to develop new products and tastes for the public palate.

The pig has always been considered to be the best and easiest option for xenotransplantation, and is considered to be closest of all our domesticated animals in biochemical terms to humans. Therefore it can be readily seen that diseases of pigs are likely to have a significant potential as zoonoses.

Ascariasis
(Large roundworm)

Infection with roundworm is estimated to affect at least 1 billion people worldwide. The intestinal nematodes of the genus *Ascaris* are common culprits. *A. lumbricoides* is usually deemed to be a human-to-human parasite transmitted by the faecal–oral route. The related worm *A. suum* is normally found in pigs; zoonotic cases have been seen. The infection is more common in areas where sanitation or hygiene routines are inadequate. Travellers to developing countries can return having been infected, as may immigrants or refugees. A previous infestation does not prevent reinfection, so patients who have been successfully treated can present with the same condition following subsequent exposure.[24]

Disease in animals

Parallel symptoms and signs are seen to human infection (see below). Migrating larvae can cause pulmonary symptoms. Symptoms of abdominal pain with diarrhoea or enteritis may be present. It is usually suckling pigs or weaners that show the worst effects. The condition is rarely fatal; however, larvae that migrate to sites other than the gut can produce unusual and severe symptoms. The cycle time from egg to adult is believed to be quicker in pigs infected with *A. suum* than it is in humans.

Transmission

Infection usually follows the ingestion of faecally contaminated raw vegetables or salad stuff carrying viable eggs. The eggs hatch in the duodenum and migrate through the gut wall and then migrate via the blood stream to the lungs.

Disease in humans

The condition may be asymptomatic or initially there may be generalised symptoms of fever and headache. Symptoms derive initially from the immune response to the infestation from either the organism itself or its metabolic products. Larvae can cause pulmonary symptoms, with asthma, pneumonia, cough and wheeze. The larvae are usually coughed up or migrate up the bronchi and are then swallowed again.

Once they return to the gut the larvae will pass through their remaining larval stages. Adults will breed in the gut; the female worm is larger than the male. Females may reach up to 35 cm in length and 4 cm in diameter. They may migrate into the biliary or pancreatic ducts. Symptoms may include gastric cramps, vomiting and diarrhoea. Pancreatitis can occur, as may intestinal obstruction and malnutrition with weight loss. Jaundice may be seen if the common bile duct is obstructed.[25,26]

The whole cycle from egg to adult takes about 2 months. Eggs passed in the faeces become infective after 2 weeks.

Some larvae may not migrate directly to the lungs and can cause complications arising from their travels or residence in the brain, eyes, liver or kidneys. The worm and its larva cause sensitisation. In some patients allergic reactions, some of which are severe, can be seen when reinfection occurs.

Diagnosis

Eggs may be identified in the stool; larvae or adults may be seen in faeces or recovered from the throat, mouth or nose. Larvae may also be present in sputum. Ultrasound, computer tomography or endoscopy may assist the diagnostic process.

Treatment

The condition may resolve without any therapeutic intervention. It is more common for anthelmintic therapy to be required.

The *BNF*[6] states that levamisole (available from IDIS Ltd) is very effective against *A. lumbricoides* and is considered to be the drug of choice. Well-tolerated, it can cause nausea and vomiting in approximately 1% of patients. A single dose of 120–150 mg in adults is normally sufficient to resolve the condition. Mebendazole may also be used at a dose of 100 mg twice daily for 3 days. Piperazine has also been used but is considered to be less suitable due to the incidence of side-effects. When used it should be given as a single dose of 4–4.5 g for adults as piperazine hydrate. Albendazole, metronidazole and pyrantel have all been used for human treatment in the USA.

Physical removal may be possible during endoscopic investigations. Larvae that migrate to sites other than the lungs during the invasive phase of development may require surgical removal. The use of anthelmintics may be associated with this migration, as it can cause larvae to flee the gut into other body organs in a random manner, leading to further complications. Early treatment of *Ascaris*-related pancreatitis usually results in complete recovery, although untreated cases can lead to a fatality rate of 3% in endemic areas.

Prevention

Vegetables and salads should be thoroughly washed before consumption to reduce or remove any contamination. Pig manure should not be used as a fertiliser or slurry on field, where produce is being actively grown.

Pasteurella
(Shipping fever, fowl cholera)

Pasteurella spp. form a group of well-recognised pathogens which are responsible for species-specific diseases. One member of the group, *P. multicocida*, has particular zoonotic potential.

Disease in animals

The organism can cause pneumonia with concurrent pleurisy in pigs, often in a mixed infection with other *Pasteurella* spp. or mycobacteria. Infected pigs are feverish and display pulmonary insufficiency, with exaggerated gasping and panting. There will often be production of blood-flecked foam from the lungs which can be seen in the mouth. Untreated cases can be fatal. A septicaemic form of the disease has also been seen in pigs and other mammals. Transmission between animals is usually by aerosol transfer.

In poultry the course of infection is very different. Turkeys, hens and other birds exhibit overwhelming diarrhoea, which is rapidly fatal in unvaccinated birds. This is normally due to *P. multicocida*, although other *Pasteurella* spp. may be present and synergistic in the disease.

Transmission

In addition to pigs and birds, many dogs, cats and horses carry *P. multicocida* as part of their oral flora, and can transmit it to other animals and humans via aerosols or saliva. These animals are often asymptomatic. Direct inoculation can occur through animal-inflicted bites or wounds. Ingestion of contaminated food or water can also lead to development of the disease.[27]

Disease in humans

Following transmission to humans there is usually localised inflammation around the infected bite or wound, followed by abscess formation and septicaemia. Pneumonia and meningitis may also occur, depending on the route of infection. In one famous case a woman developed meningitis after kissing her dog, although it is likely that she was at enhanced risk because of her concurrent gingivitis.[28]

Infection by this organism is a serious risk, particularly to children, who tend to receive more bites from companion animals in rough play, the elderly and the immunocompromised, where infection can be rapidly progressive and fatal. Septicaemic forms have been seen in patients who are suffering from HIV/AIDS or liver cirrhosis or who are on chemotherapy regimes.

The disease is notifiable, and the PHLS receives on average notification of approximately 200 cases annually, usually following bite injuries.

Treatment

Antibiotic therapy at standard therapeutic doses is normally sufficient to cure the condition, although in more serious cases supportive treatment may also be required. The drugs of choice are the tetracyclines, penicillins or cephalosporins: length of course and dosages are linked to age, weight, drug allergies and clinical response in the normal manner.

Prevention

Wounds, especially those inflicted by animals, must be thoroughly and rapidly cleansed and disinfected. Companion animals should not be allowed to lick patients' faces or wounds. Encouraging children to wash their hands and, if necessary, faces after playing with or touching animals is an important preventive measure. Vaccination is available and widely used in pigs and poultry to lower the incidence of the disease. Those involved in equestrian pursuits should recognise that bites from horses pose a particular threat from this organism.

Streptococcus suis

Disease in animals

Streptococcus suis is a pathogenic streptococcus, found in pigs. The type 2 serotype is usually responsible for severe disease in swine, and also for the occasional cases seen in humans. Infection is often inapparent; however, in clinical cases it can cause pneumonia, septicaemia, septic arthritis and meningitis with behavioural changes, fever, and ultimately paralysis. Infections in herds of swine can result in high rates of mortality.

Transmission

Transmission to humans follows the handling of infected meat or carcasses, and it is therefore no surprise that most of the 34 cases reported between 1982 and 1998 to the PHLS occurred in abattoir workers, meat handlers, farm workers or veterinary surgeons. The annual case rate in humans is usually in low single figures; the disease is notifiable under the Notification of Infectious Diseases System (NOIDS) and Reporting of Injuries, Diseases, and Dangerous Occurrences Regulations (RIDDOR), and also animal health legislation, so it is included for completeness.

Disease in humans

In humans the pathogen causes fever and, very occasionally, meningitis. Residual deafness has been reported in patients after the infection has resolved.

Diagnosis

Diagnosis is confirmed by culturing the organism or using PCR assay. Treatment is usually initiated before identification.

Treatment

Treatment is usually oral penicillins or erythromycin with monitoring as to efficacy, as resistant serotypes have been identified in mainland Europe.

Prevention

Prevention revolves around good hygiene procedures and the use of protective clothing. All wounds should be covered and any occurring during handling of meat or carcasses should be disinfected thoroughly and dressed swiftly.

Trichinosis

This condition is caused by a tissue nematode of the family *Trichinella*. In the past most cases were associated with *T. spiralis*, but recently there have been cases of *T. pseudospiralis* causing human disease.

The parasite is normally associated with pigs and dogs. Rats, cats and certain wild animals are also capable of acting as zoonotic reservoirs. It is an affliction that is worldwide in its distribution.[29, 30]

Disease in animals

Pigs fed on offal or swill containing animal tissue which has not been sufficiently heat-treated are at the greatest risk of contracting the disease, although there have been recorded cases following pigs eating the corpses of rats. The number of human cases seen in western countries has been dramatically reduced by changes in feeding practice for pigs, and by meat inspection. A group of cases of *T. pseudospiralis* in 1999 was related to the ingestion of wild boar meat in the Camargue area of France.[31]

Encysted larval stages are ingested in animal tissue and then hatch in the gut of the host; these then develop into adults in the surface layers of the intestine. Eggs are produced by the female worms, and these worms hatch to produce larvae. The larvae pass through the intestinal wall and penetrate into the associated lymphatic or venous blood vessels. They can then be distributed around the rest of the body of the host and will normally encyst in muscle tissue as a result of the host's immune response. The cysts may become calcified over time and can be detected in the muscle. The fibres of the muscle may be torn or damaged by the invasion of the parasite. The affected animal normally displays no clinical signs of infection. Infection with *T. pseudospiralis* does not evoke the same immune response and the cyst wall is normally not present.

Transmission

As with other mammals, infection in humans follows the ingestion of infected animal tissue.

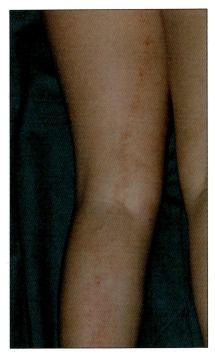

Plate 1 Cutaneous larva migrans: a linear skin rash on a child's leg caused by the burrowing larvae of nematode hookworms (*Ancylostoma* spp.). Courtesy of Dr P. Marazzi (Science Photo Library).

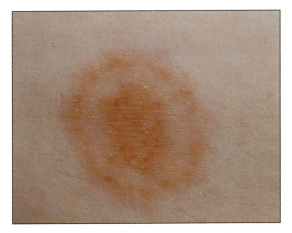

Plate 2 Ringworm lesion. Courtesy of Science Photo Library.

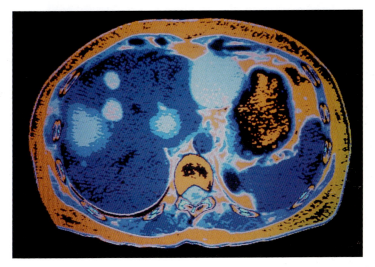

Plate 3 Hydatid disease. Coloured computed tomography scan showing cysts (light areas) in the liver (blue, left) due to hydatid disease. This is a horizontal slice through the abdomen with the patient's back at the bottom of the picture. At lower centre is the spine (pale blue), at right the spleen (blue) and stomach (orange). Courtesy of GJLP-CNRI/Science Photo Library.

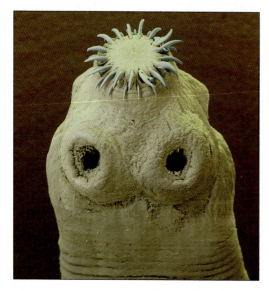

Plate 4 Light micrograph of the scolex of a parasitic tapeworm, *Taenia taeniformis*. The scolex has hooklets and suckers (circular), by which the worm attaches itself to the intestines of its host. Courtesy of Eye of Science/Science Photo Library.

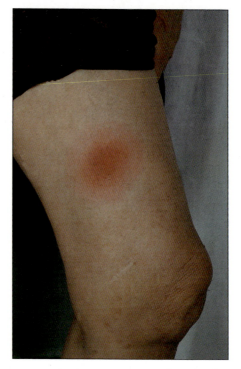

Plate 5 Erythema migrans rash (Lyme disease). Courtesy of Larry Mulvehill/Science Photo Library.

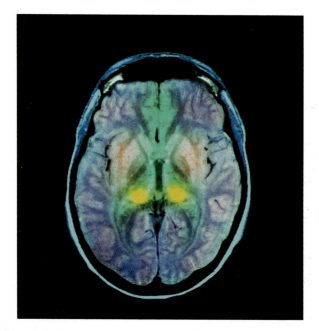

Plate 6 Creutzfeldt–Jakob disease (CJD). Coloured magnetic resonance imaging (MRI) scan of the brain of a 17-year-old male suffering from CJD (new variant) in 1997. In this axial slice through the brain, the folded cerebrum is seen forming two hemispheres. At lower centre are two yellow areas of the thalamus, diseased with CJD. It is detected as a bilateral signal abnormality on MRI. Courtesy of Simon Fraser/Royal Victoria Infirmary, Newcastle upon Tyne/Science Photo Library.

Disease in humans

The severity of symptoms displayed is proportional to the number of viable encysted larvae ingested. The mildest cases are usually subclinical with perhaps a small amount of muscle soreness being present. In heavy infestations there may be an abrupt onset of muscle pain, fever and swelling of the eyelids, followed by haemorrhages in the retina, conjunctiva and mouth with associated pain. An aversion to bright light (photophobia) may also occur. The most commonly seen sites for larvae to encyst are the diaphragm, ribs, biceps, larynx, tongue and jaw or neck muscles. This may lead to difficulties in chewing and swallowing.

As the infection progresses patients may display a profound thirst, with profuse sweating. There may be gastrointestinal disturbance with diarrhoea, stomach cramps and nausea. In 10–20% of patients showing severe symptoms there may be progression to cardiac, renal or central nervous system involvement. Fatalities due to myocardial failure have been recorded. Provided that patients do not succumb to the condition, it is normal for a complete recovery to be made over a period of months, although there may be residual damage with sequelae.

Diagnosis

Diagnosis is made using serological testing or muscle biopsy. ELISA and PCR methods can be used successfully.

Treatment

Most cases resolve spontaneously, so purely symptomatic treatment and support is necessary. The *BNF*[6] makes no recommendations, and specialist help would be necessary in treating the disease. In the USA, tiabendazole anthelmintics such as mebendazole, tiabendazole or albendazole have been used to treat the condition. There is evidence, however, that once an infection is established these drugs only eliminate the adults and larvae in the gut, and prevent further egg and larval production, leaving any migrating or tissue-dwelling larvae intact. Corticosteroids have been used to control the systemic inflammation caused by migrating larvae. The patients in the French case cluster of *T. pseudospiralis* were treated with albendazole at a rate of 800 mg/day for 10 days combined with prednisolone at a dosage of 30 mg/kg per day for the first 3 days.

Prevention

Ensuring that all swill or offal fed to pigs has been thoroughly heated at greater than 77°C prevents infection by ingestion of any infected animal tissue. Rats should be controlled in pig units and general hygiene measures, including the isolation and removal of sick individuals, should be enforced. There may be an issue relating to organic methods of pig rearing, and the possibility of infection being acquired from wild sources. This is also true of herds of domesticated or semidomesticated boar, now extensively bred for meat in outdoor conditions. As *T. pseudospiralis* has now been identified as a possible human pathogen, there are some concerns that current meat inspection methods which are geared to the detection of encysted forms may not be sufficient, as this species does not evoke cyst formation response from the afflicted host. If more cases arise, there may be a need for alternative methods of detection.

Meat should be carefully inspected, and pork should be thoroughly cooked so as to reach more than 77°C in the centre. Suspect meat can also be rendered safe by prolonged freezing for more than 3 weeks.

Miscellaneous agricultural zoonoses

The keeping of animals as a production process has always been traditionally part of agricultural enterprise. Over the last few decades this has been extended to certain animals that were previously seen on the menu after they had been hunted and killed in the wild, or on managed country estates. To satisfy demand for the more unusual, farming of salmon and deer for the table has become an important industry.

The following two diseases relate to deer. Lyme disease is endemic in certain areas in the UK, and poses a threat to people exposed to the causative spirochaete *Borrelia burgdorferi*. The second condition, tularaemia, has not been detected in the UK but it is endemic in the rest of western Europe, and the Pet Travel Scheme (PETS) passport regulations insist that animals licensed under the scheme should be treated for ectoparasites to prevent Lyme disease as well as other tick- and flea-borne diseases.

Lyme disease
(Tick-borne borreliosis)

Lyme disease is caused by spirochaetes of various *Borrelia* spp. The disease is named after the town of Lyme, Connecticut, USA, where a cluster of juvenile arthritis cases in the 1970s were first linked to infection by *B. burgdorferi*. Studies of collected insects and literature surveys on both sides of the Atlantic have identified the organism and the disease was clinically described in the late 19th century.[32]

Transmission

The infection is transmitted by the bite of an *Ixodes* tick, mainly *I. scapularis* or *I. dammini* in North America, which normally preys on deer. In the UK *I. ricinus* has been identified as the main tick vector and infectious reservoir. *Ixodes* spp. ticks are much smaller than common dog or cattle ticks. In their larval and nymphal stages they are no bigger than a pinhead. Adult ticks are slightly larger. Other biting insects, such as mosquitoes and fleas, have also been implicated in transmission, but they are not believed to be an infectious reservoir. Rather they are an incidental vector infected by feeding on an infected vertebrate.

Incidence

Reported incidents of Lyme disease have risen in England and Wales in recent years. This probably arises from better recognition of the disease and more thorough reporting. Incidence and prevalence are related to environmental factors. Certain weather conditions, such as drought or high rainfall, can kill the tick before maturation.[33]

In England and Wales, surveillance by the PHLS has demonstrated the infection in 68 counties. The main affected areas are Hampshire, Wiltshire and Dorset, linked to foci in the New Forest and Salisbury Plain. Devon, Somerset and Norfolk have a higher-than-average incidence of cases. The PHLS has also identified that many of the cases reported in the UK have been acquired abroad, mainly in the USA, France, Germany, Austria and Scandinavia. There were 162 cases of Lyme disease reported to the PHLS in 1998. The annual figure has increased over the last decade, probably reflecting greater awareness of the disease, rather than greater incidence.[33]

Life cycle

The life cycle of the tick and the *Borrelia* spp. are closely linked. The female tick lays eggs during the spring of the first year. These hatch into larvae in early summer. The larvae then seek out rodents and birds as hosts. These hosts, being highly mobile, help disseminate the tick over a wider geographical area. The larvae continue to feed over the summer and become dormant in the autumn. The following spring the larvae moult into nymphs which attach themselves to small rodents and other small mammals. In the autumn of the second year they moult again into adults. At this time ticks will attach to a large mammalian host, feeding persistently and mating. The female will then drop off and lay her eggs, starting the cycle again (Figure 3.1).

The *Borrelia* spp. are present in all stages of the tick, acquiring the infection from infected rodents when feeding commences. As the larvae are the most voracious and aggressive feeders, these actively spread the organism. This correlates with the incidence of infection. Most tick bites which lead to clinical manifestations occur in the period May to July

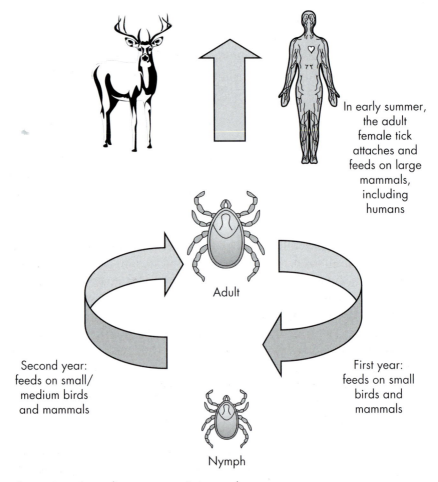

In early summer, the adult female tick attaches and feeds on large mammals, including humans

Adult

Second year: feeds on small/ medium birds and mammals

First year: feeds on small birds and mammals

Nymph

Figure 3.1 Lyme disease: transmission cycle.

when the larvae and nymphal stages are actively biting. Deer are the preferred host; humans, cats and dogs are incidental hosts, as are cattle and horses. Dogs suffer badly from the arthritic form of the disease.

Disease in humans

In humans, as with other spirochaetal diseases, the course of the disease is undulant, with acute and chronic phases interspersed with long asymptomatic periods. After the initial manifestation there can be a latent period of up to 4 years before further clinical signs are seen.[34]

Initial infection follows a tick bite; it is now believed that the tick must stay attached for a period for transmission to occur. This period can be less than 16 hours: 24–72 hours is believed to give optimal transmission. A localised skin reaction appeared in 60% of English cases.[33] This occurs at the bite site, usually about 9 days after infection due to spirochaetal invasion. This is called erythema migrans. It presents as an expanding reddened area (Plate 5). It usually has reinforced borders and can be solid or annular. It may be warm to touch but rarely is itchy or painful.

Later some patients will have flu-like symptoms with fever, malaise and headache. A transient lymphadenopathy may be seen, as may organ involvement with transient hepatitis. Eye problems, including conjunctivitis or optic nerve damage, have been reported.[35] A widespread erythema migrans with multiple lesions can occur, often in conjunction with other more serious symptoms of neurological damage, cardiac involvement or arthritis. A condition called acrodermatitis chronica atrophicans (ACA) is occasionally seen. It is a serious condition, passing from an initial inflammatory stage into atrophy and pigmentation disturbances of the skin on extensor surfaces of the limbs. Accompanying symptoms include pain, itching and paraesthesia.

Neurological complications may manifest at any time: 24% of UK patients under 14 years of age suffer some neurological symptoms. This falls to 14% in other age groups. Symptoms range from meningitis, cranial nerve damage and facial palsy to peripheral neuropathies. Subarachnoid haemorrhage and seizures have also been reported. A chronic form of the disease with memory loss, loss of motor skills and dementia is reported, although the linkage to *Borrelia* infection is currently unproven.[36]

Up to 10% of infected individuals in the USA present with associated cardiac problems. These include atrioventricular block, heart failure and myocarditis that resolves on treatment with antimicrobials.[37]

In the USA it is estimated that 14% of sufferers develop arthritis, although in none of the cases linked to the New Forest in the UK was any arthritis seen.[33] The first symptoms may appear 3–6 weeks after first infection, usually with a single joint involvement, commonly the knee. The jaw, ankles, shoulders, elbows and wrists are also common sites.[38]

The variation in symptoms seen between the USA and the UK seems to be related to a difference in the genospecies of the pathogen. In the USA *B. burgdorferi* predominates, whereas in Europe, *B. afzelii* and *B. garinii* are more common. Different clinical manifestations are species-related, with *B. afzelii* being associated with dermatological symptoms and *B. garinii* with neurological disorders.

Treatment

Treatment consists solely of antibiotic therapy. Patients with severe multisystemic involvement, especially where neurological symptoms are present, can be treated with intravenous cephalosporins. Tetracyclines, especially doxycycline, and penicillins, particularly amoxicillin, demonstrate efficacy against most *Borrelia* infections. Beta-lactams are relatively inefficient and should only be used when other agents are not suitable.[39]

Prevention

Prevention strategies can be divided into environmental and personal. Many prevention regimes aim to break the ability of the organism to maintain a rodent reservoir, and prevent tick attachment to large mammals or humans. Controlling undergrowth around footpaths and inspecting and treating livestock for ticks can reduce the tick population. Controlling access of rodents to commercially farmed deer can reduce infection risks both for animals and for associated human workers.

Personal protection, especially for individuals employed in forestry or other business in endemic areas, consists of wearing long trousers and boots, with the trousers tucked into the socks. Lighter-coloured clothing allows ticks to be spotted before they can establish a potentially infective bite. Prompt removal of any ticks is also important, and examining the groin, armpits and scalp is particularly important. Outdoor enthusiasts should take similar precautions, especially if camping in areas where ticks are known to be endemic.[40]

Tularaemia
(Francis' disease, deer-fly fever, rabbit fever, O'Hara disease)

Tularaemia is caused by *Francisella tularensis*, a small Gram-negative coccobacillus. An intracellular pathogen, it can also survive in the environment for extended periods. It has now been found to be able to parasitise life forms as lowly as amoebae and other protozoans. The organism is named after Sir Edward Francis who initially isolated and studied the causative organism at Tulare in California, USA. It appears to exist in two types or biovars, classified as types A or B. Classification of the organism relates to the comparative virulence or pathogenicity and the two types seem to have different geographical ranges. Type A is found mostly in the USA and possesses particular affinity and pathogenicity for humans and rabbits but is also found in many other mammalian species as well as ticks and biting flies. Type B bacteria are found in the USA, Europe and Asia with less affinity for humans and more for aquatic mammals.

Francisella spp. appear to produce an endotoxin similar to those produced by other Gram-negative enteric bacilli. An additional twist to the organism is that *F. tularensis* has also been suggested as a possible agent for biological terrorism or warfare. There is some evidence that Israel and Russia have attempted to develop resistant strains for use as weapons.

The organism can also survive in water and penetrate intact skin. As the estimate of inoculum necessary to initiate disease in humans has been set at only 10 organisms, the disease is classified as highly infective. Although not reported in the UK, with the increasing popularity of adventure holidays where trekking or living in wilderness areas forms part of the itinerary, there is a risk of exposure and disease for tourists who might then return home before clinical signs are seen.

Recent outbreaks include one in Kosovo in May 2000. Of 724 suspected cases, 306 were confirmed as type B tularaemia, and were linked to rodents. Spread to humans was linked to rat-associated ticks, fleas or lice as vectors. There were no cases in peace-keeping or aid workers and no fatalities, as all cases resolved on treatment. Slovakia first recorded the disease in 1985; Austria has recorded 418 cases in the period 1985–1998. In Austria, the Czech Republic and Slovakia, outbreaks have been linked to small mammals and their associated ticks as a reservoir for the disease.

In the Former Soviet Union routine vaccination is carried out, as the disease appears to be endemic, with 1485 cases being recorded in sporadic outbreaks between 1992 and 1999. Of these cases, 70% appeared in urban populations, with 30% in children. In 1998 an outbreak occurred in Sweden, with 81 confirmed cases. There have also been outbreaks as far apart as Bulgaria between 1998 and 2000 and Spain, where 24 cases were recorded between January and April 2000. In many of these outbreaks a small and increasing number of cases were seen over a period of time, reaching a peak in incidence and then declining. The same pattern has been seen in the USA where the disease was very prevalent in the 1950s but has decreased markedly over time, with sporadic outbreaks now occurring.

It is not known why the incidence has declined but the use of insecticides, changes in agricultural practice and habitat destruction have all been suggested as factors. Outbreaks such as the Kosovan incident may be associated with boom years for the population of vermin hosts such as rabbits or rats, and thus the blood-sucking parasite population.

The prevalence of the disease shows a marked seasonal bias related, as with Lyme disease, to the life cycle of the ticks that can be the main vector for its spread in certain areas. Most cases reported between May and October are associated with parasite bites. Another peak is seen in the winter relating to hunting, where there is no vector spread but there is direct contact between humans and animals during the skinning and preparation of prey animals. This may explain why most cases are seen in adult males – over 75% of American cases are seen in male hunters.

The reservoir for the disease consists of both wild and domestic animals. It has been found in rabbits, hares, squirrels, deer, snakes, rodents, cats, dogs, cattle, pigs, sheep and goats. The organism has also been isolated from all the life stages of various ticks, and *Dermacentor reticulatus* (dog tick) and *Ixodes ricinus* (castor oil bean tick) are the major European species involved. The organism can persist for many months or years in the tissues of the tick and is carried through moults and can be transferred from mother to offspring. The organism has been isolated from tick saliva and faecal matter, so inoculation of a wound with either substance can provide sufficient inoculum to produce clinical disease. Luckily, not all ticks within a population are infected. Mosquitoes, deer and horseflies and fleas have also been found to carry the organism. Whether they are competent vectors of transfer is not proven in all species, although in the USA deer flies are known to be a major vector. It has also been demonstrated that cats are able to transmit the bacterium on their claws, after catching infected prey.[41]

Disease in animals

In animals, the main clinical manifestation of the disease is septicaemia, with high fever, stiffness and loss of appetite. Respiratory involvement may also manifest with symptoms similar to pleurisy. Death follows frequently and rapidly. On autopsy, necrotic lesions may be found in the main organs.

Transmission

Humans are susceptible to infection with the organism and it can affect any age group or social group.

Infection in humans follows a vector bite, physical contact with an infected animal or an ingested inoculum from water or meat. Human-to-human spread does not occur. As has been previously stated, the organism can also penetrate intact skin.

Disease in humans

Following infection there is a prepatent period of 2–10 days before clinical signs are seen. An ulcer appears at the inoculation site and local lymph gland swelling is seen in the lymph nodes nearest to the ulcer as the organism multiplies and proliferates. Initially there may be a high fever, which then subsides and recurs in a cyclic manner. Chills, headache, malaise, anorexia and fatigue are quite common.

Antibody production begins during the second or third week of infection but is usually insufficient to protect against infection.

The disease presents in a variety of forms depending on the route of infection. The Centers for Disease Control and Prevention classification in the USA recognises six main forms: glandular, ulceroglandular, oculoglandular, oropharyngeal, pneumonic and typhoidal. The classification is useful; however, the clinical symptoms associated with various forms of the disease often present at the same time in the same patient, leading to confusion. The mortality rate for untreated tularaemia is about 8%; early diagnosis and treatment can reduce that rate to below 1%.

The most common type, seen in over 75% of cases, is classified as ulceroglandular following cutaneous inoculation. When the initial ulcers are seen, their location may help to identify the mode of transmission. Ulcers on the upper limbs usually result from exposure to infected animals, whereas ulcers on the lower limbs, back or abdomen usually result from parasitic bites. Glandular swelling follows appearance of the ulcer, with primary sites again related to mode of transmission. Untreated ulcers can take a long time to heal, with associated persistent lymph node swellings. Most cases will take 3–5 weeks to resolve without treatment; however, symptoms can persist for up to 3 years after the appearance of the disease. Many cases will need a lengthy period of convalescence.[42]

The glandular form presents in a similar manner to the ulceroglandular disease but without skin ulceration and is responsible for 15–20% of the cases in the USA. Glandular involvement can be acute and severe.

Fortunately, the oculoglandular type of infection is rare. It occurs in no more than 4% of cases in most outbreaks and less than 1% over a series of outbreaks, although it may appear in single case occurrences where there is only one individual infected. Infected material, for instance, blood, meat, dust or bodily fluids, is splashed into the eye. Following infection the eyelids swell and there is ulceration in the conjunctiva and surface of the eyeball. Localised glandular swelling in the neck may also be present.

Ingestion of contaminated meat or water can lead to the oropharyngeal form. In recent outbreaks, 4–18% of cases have presented with sore throat and pharyngitis. In some individuals, the throat does not appear to be infected on examination. Others show severe inflammation with involvement of the tonsils and swelling to nearly total closure. Swelling is seen in the glands of the jaw, throat and neck.

The pneumonic form follows inhalation of infected aerosols; the symptoms and findings in this form vary. As in the other forms, fever and glandular swellings are usually present. Lung involvement may mimic a chest infection or pleurisy.

The last in the list of forms is the typhoidal type. Onset is usually abrupt and follows ingestion of infected material. High fever is seen, with aching joints and muscles, vomiting and diarrhoea. Liver and splenic enlargement is sometimes seen, and usually develops gradually after the acute phase. Skin rashes may also be present.

In all types of infection, some of which will fall into one or more categories, long-term immunity will usually follow infection.

Diagnosis

Confirming a diagnosis is made using clinical samples. The organism is difficult to culture in a laboratory, and also poses a risk to laboratory personnel. Immunofluorescence or PCR methods and serological testing are preferable, and recent advances have been made in producing rapid reliable test methods.

Treatment

The treatment of tularaemia depends on rapid diagnosis and the commencement of antibiotic therapy as soon as possible after clinical signs are seen. Antibiotic use is the only therapy, using single or combination therapy.

Streptomycin with or without the addition of a tetracycline has historically been the mainstay of treatment. Chloramphenicol has been substituted for tetracycline on occasions, although the side-effects associated with chloramphenicol make it less than desirable. Streptomycin is usually given intramuscularly at a dose of 30–40 mg/kg per day in two divided doses for a duration of 7 days. An alternative regime is 40 mg/kg per day in two divided doses for 3 days followed by a period of 4 days at half the previous dose twice daily. Gentamicin has been substituted for streptomycin in a dosage of 6 mg/kg per day by intravenous infusion every 8 hours for 7–14 days, with the length of the course being linked to patient response. Clinical monitoring of blood chemistry is essential with the use of these aminoglycosides.[43]

Tetracyclines are effective, but as they are bacteriostatic rather than bactericidal, the duration of therapy needs to be longer. Doxycycline is given by mouth at a dosage of 100 mg every 12 hours for 10–14 days. Some studies have shown that high-dose erythromycin is suitable for type A infections; however, the type B serotype is known to be resistant. In a recent outbreak in Sweden the 4-quinolones were used. Ciprofloxacin was given by mouth for 10–14 days at a dosage of 15–20 mg/kg daily in two divided doses in children under 10, and at a dosage of 1000–1500 mg daily in two divided doses to adults and children over 10. Norfloxacin 400 mg/day in divided doses for 12 days was used in a single patient in the same outbreakand proved effective. Both ciprofloxacin and doxycycline have the advantage of allowing community treatment as they can be effectively given by mouth rather than requiring an injection programme and the use of secondary healthcare resources.[44]

Prevention

A vaccine is available for people considered to be at high risk or where the disease is seen as a public health issue, such as in the Former Soviet

Union. Vaccination has also been used where the disease is a possible health and safety hazard of employment, for example in park rangers and field naturalists in endemic areas. The main human groups at risk of occupational exposure are farmers, shepherds, hunters, veterinary surgeons, meat handlers, cooks and the partners of hunters.

Prevention is the best policy. Avoiding insect bites and implementing hygiene procedures when living or travelling in areas where there is a high prevalence of the disease are essential measures. Use of insecticides and wearing suitable clothing in forested areas – trousers rather than shorts – will prevent many tick bites. Any ticks which succeed in attaching should be removed carefully without crushing them, and whenever possible not with bare hands. Domestic animals suffering from the disease should be treated or culled to prevent spread.

As with leptospirosis, drinking, washing or swimming either by choice or accidentally in infected water should be avoided wherever possible. Hunters and others who handle or butcher wild animals should be advised to wear suitable protective clothing. Wild game should be thoroughly cooked, and as the organism can survive prolonged freezing, suitable precautions should be taken when handling any raw game meat. Antibiotic prophylaxis is not recommended in any risk group.

Zoonoses of feral and wild animals

Not all of the animals encountered in the UK, or elsewhere, fall neatly into either companion or domestic categories. Some will be animals, once domesticated, which have returned to wild living. These feral species are especially important infective reservoirs not only for zoonoses, but also for other significant animal diseases. Some animals have never been domesticated, and will be wild. Some will inhabit only rural or wilderness areas; others will have adapted their mode of survival to living in or around the encroaching urban environment. There are probably now more urban foxes in our towns and cities than there are in the countryside.

Feral and wild animals generally suffer the diseases associated with their closest domesticated relatives. In the case of feral species the difference between them and domesticated animals is solely a matter of geography, and many are escapees, such as racing pigeons. The large flocks of pigeons encountered in urban centres have been implicated as a reservoir for *Chlamydia psittaci*, and cause a significant nuisance. There may also be ornamental or exotic introductions which have managed to evade control, for example muntjac deer, coypu or edible dormice. Cats and, to a far smaller extent, dogs can live a feral existence and are usually reservoirs of the afflictions of their own species, which may not be zoonoses.

Wild animals such as foxes, badgers, rats and squirrels also have their own associated diseases. Badgers as a reservoir of tuberculosis are of particular concern, although the scientific evidence relating to transmission into cattle is conflicting. Foxes are on the increase, and as they become more established in urban areas, they form a potential reservoir for canine zoonoses, especially as they not only hunt but also scavenge, and consumption of other mammalian corpses is a potential route of spread in certain infections. Rodents as a reservoir for leptospirosis are well recognised, and the emergence of animals resistant to the rodenticides in normal widespread use poses an increasing problem, especially in urban areas. The need to control populations of pest animals and their associated arthropod or intestinal parasites in urban areas is a significant part of the agenda to maintain environmental and public health.

Good agricultural practice includes reducing mammalian pest species. This has become less routine due to the costs involved and the concerns of the environmental lobby. Control of pests on and around farms is vitally important in the prevention and control of spread of certain zoonoses. It becomes even more significant when the pest and the domesticated species are very closely related; sparrows in a chicken run, or in the feed mill associated with such a unit, would pose a significant risk for avian disease transfer.

Most feral or wild animals shun human contact; therefore direct zoonotic transmission is unlikely outside specialist sanctuaries or rescue units. The majority of these units have standing procedures under which all animals are treated as suspect and as possible biohazards, thus preventing untoward incidents of injury or infective transfer.

Members of the public should be encouraged to be circumspect in their handling of injured wild animals, and children should be educated not to touch corpses of birds or mammals. Normal hygiene routines should be observed, with the use of protective clothing and general hygiene measures. In the event of any injury caused by a wild animal, medical attention should be sought as soon as reasonably practicable.

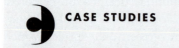

CASE STUDIES

Case study 3

Mr and Mrs Evans are a semiretired couple in their late 40s. They are well-known for booking holidays from the last-minute bargains on Teletext. Mr Evans has very forthright views on immunisation and malaria prophylaxis, which he considers to be a waste of time and money. 'If I am going to catch something nasty, I will catch it anyway' is a phrase you have learnt to associate with him.

In early January, Mr and Mrs Evans decide some winter sun is in order and book a bargain break to Goa. After their return Mr Evans complains of a small red lump on his foot near his toes. This has started to migrate slowly across his foot and is causing some irritation. Within a week it has reached the ankle bone and is starting to move upward.

Mrs Evans meanwhile has had episodic diarrhoea. This has been treated with loperamide and metoclopramide as she is also getting bouts of nausea. Despite the treatment, the condition is persistent and Mrs Evans is complaining of abdominal distension with large amounts of evil-smelling gas being expelled, especially when she has the bouts of diarrhoea.

Questions
1. What is the likely cause for Mr Evans's condition?
2. What are the available treatment options?
3. How could it have been prevented?
4. What is the likely cause of Mrs Evans's condition?
5. What aspects of her condition support this diagnosis, and how would it be confirmed?
6. What is the most likely treatment agent?

Case study 4

Mr Figgis is an old friend. His son Michael has been camping out in the New Forest for his Duke of Edinburgh award scheme. When you next meet Mr Figgis in the street he informs you that Michael has been slightly unwell since his return from the last camping trip.

He tells you Michael had a tick attached to his forehead when he returned and that, although he took Michael to the surgery, the general practitioner removed the tick but prescribed no drugs. Since then Michael has had a transient rash around the bite, and has been complaining of feeling hot and cold with shivering fits. Mr Figgis has put this down to a slight chill, and then starts talking about how bad the weather has been for his begonias.

Questions
1. What is the condition Michael could be suffering from?
2. What signs or symptoms support this diagnosis?
3. What is the best treatment?
4. Why is it particularly important that Michael is treated now?

References

1. Trott D G, Pilsworth R. Outbreaks of conjunctivitis due to the Newcastle disease virus among workers in chicken-broiler factories. *BMJ* 1965; 25: 1514–1517.
2. Amato Gauci A J. The return of brucellosis. *Maltese Med J* 1995; 7: 7–8.
3. Corbel M J. Brucellosis: an overview. *Emerg Infect Dis* 1997; 3: 213–221.
4. Mantur B G, Mangalgi S S, Mulimani B. *Brucella melitensis* – a sexually transmissible agent. *Lancet* 1996; 347: 1763.
5. Santini C, Baiocchi P, Berardelli A, *et al*. A case of brain abscess due to *Brucella melitensis*. *Clin Infect Dis* 1994; 19: 977–978.
6. Mehta DK, ed. *British National Formulary*, vol. 42. London: British Medical Association/Royal Pharmaceutical Society of Great Britain, 2001.
7. Bauer K. Foot-and-mouth disease as a zoonosis. *Arch Virol* 1997; 13 (suppl.): 95–97.
8. Prempeh H, Smith R, Muller B. Foot-and-mouth disease: the human consequences. *BMJ* 2001; 322: 565–566.
9. World Health Organization. *Foot and Mouth Disease: Consequences for Public Health*. WHO (CSR), 2001. http://www.who.int/emc/surveill/index.html
10. Maurin M, Raoult D. Q fever. *Clin Microbiol Rev* 1999; 12: 518–553.
11. Raoult D, Tissot-Dupont H, Foucault C, *et al*. Q fever 1985–1998: clinical and epidemiologic features of 1383 infections. *Medicine (Baltimore)* 2000; 79: 109–123.
12. Lowinger-Seoane M, Torres-Rodriguez J M, Madrenys-Brunet N, *et al*. Extensive dermatophytoses caused by *Trichophyton mentagrophytes* and *Microsporum canis* in a patient with AIDS. *Mycopathologia* 1992; 120: 143–146.
13. Evans C, Garcia H H, Gilman R H, Friedland J S. Controversies in the management of cysticercosis. *Emerg Infect Dis* 1997; 3: 403–405.
14. Salinas R, Prasad K. Drugs for treating neurocysticercosis (tapeworm infection of the brain) (Cochrane review). *Cochrane Library* 2001, 2. http://www.update-software.com/Cochrane
15. Daborn C J, Grange J M: HIV/AIDS and its implication for the control of animal tuberculosis. *Br Vet J* 1993; 149: 405–417.
16. Weltman A C, Rose D N. The safety of Bacille Calmette-Guérin vaccination in HIV infection and AIDS. *AIDS* 1993; 7: 149–157.
17. Villemonteix P, Agius G, Ducroz B, *et al*. Pregnancy complicated by severe *Chlamydia psittaci* infection acquired from a goat flock: a case report. *Eur J Obstet Gynecol Reprod Biol* 1990; 37: 91–94.
18. Daniel M, Jorgensen D M. Gestational psittacosis in a Montana sheep rancher. *Emerg Infect Dis* 1997; 3: 191–194.
19. Hill D R. Giardiasis, issues in diagnosis and management. *Infect Dis Clin North Am* 1993; 7: 503–525.
20. Lengerich E J, Addiss D G, Juranek D D. Severe giardiasis in the United States. *Clin Infect Dis* 1994; 18: 760–763.
21. Wittner M, Tanowitz H, Weiss L. Parasitic infections in AIDS patients. *Infect Dis Clin North Am* 1993; 7: 569–586.
22. Robinson A J, Petersen G V. Orf virus infection of workers in the meat industry. *N Z Med J* 1983; 96: 81–85.

23. Health and Safety Executive. *Common Zoonoses in Agriculture* 12/96. Agricultural Information Sheet AIS2(rev). Sudbury, Suffolk: Health and Safety Executive, 1996.

24. Shad J A, Lee Y A. Pancreatitis due to *Ascaris lumbricoides*: second occurrence after 2 years. *South Med J* 2001; 94: 78–80.

25. Sandouk F, Haffar S, Zada M, *et al.* Pancreatic-biliary ascariasis: experience of 300 cases. *Am J Gastroenterol* 1997; 92: 2264–2267.

26. Maddern G J, Dennison A R, Blumgart L H. Fatal *Ascaris* pancreatitis: an uncommon problem in the west. *Gut* 1992; 33: 402–403.

27. Francis D P, Holmes M A, Brandon G. *Pasteurella multocida*, infections after domestic animal bites and scratches. *JAMA* 1975; 233: 42–45.

28. Drabick J J, Gasser R A, Saunders N B, *et al. Pasteurella multocida* pneumonia in a man with AIDS and nontraumatic feline exposure. *Chest* 1993; 103: 7–11.

29. Andrews J R H, Ainsworth R, Pozio E. Nematodes in human muscle. *Parasitol Today* 1997; 13: 488–489.

30. Jongwutiwes S, Chantachum N, Kraivichian P, *et al.* First outbreak of human trichinellosis caused by *Trichinella pseudospiralis*. *Clin Infect Dis* 1998; 26: 111–115.

31. Ranque S, Faugere B, Pozio E, *et al. Trichinella pseudospiralis* outbreak in France. *Emerg Infect Dis* 2000; 6 online: htttp://www.cdc.gov/ncidod/eid/index.htm

32. Hubband M J, Baker A S, Carr K J. Distribution of *Borrelia burgdorferi* s.l. spirochaete DNA in British ticks (*Argasidae* and *Ixodidae*) since 19th century assessed by PCR. *Med Vet Entomol* 1998; 12: 89–97.

33. Smith R, O'Connell S, Palmer S. Lyme disease surveillance in England and Wales 1986–1998. *Emerg Infect Dis* 2000; 6: 4.

34. Cutler S J. Lyme borreliosis: an update. *Br J Hosp Med.* 1996; 56: 581–584.

35. Lesser R L. Ocular manifestations of Lyme disease. *Am J Med* 1995; 98: 60S–62S.

36. Chehrenama M, Zagardo M T, Koski C L. Subarachnoid hemorrhage in a patient with Lyme disease. *Neurology* 1997; 48: 520–523.

37. McAlister H F, Klementowicz P T, Andrews C, *et al.* Lyme carditis: an important cause of reversible heart block. *Ann Intern Med* 1989; 110: 339–345.

38. Steere A C. Diagnosis and treatment of Lyme arthritis. *Med Clin North Am* 1997; 81: 179–194.

39. Kuna E, Volkman D J. Therapeutic options for the treatment of Lyme disease. *Infect Med* 1993; 10: 38–44.

40. Couch P, Johnson C E. Prevention of Lyme disease. *Am J Hosp Pharm* 1992; 49: 1164–1173.

41. Cepellan J, Fong I W. Tularemia from a cat bite: case report and review of feline-associated tularemia. *Clin Infect Dis* 1993; 16: 472–475.

42. Cerny Z. Skin manifestations of tularemia. *Int J Dermatol* 1994; 33: 468–470.

43. Enderlin G, Morales L, Jacobs R F, *et al.* Streptomycin and alternative agents for the treatment of tularemia: review of the literature. *Clin Infect Dis* 1994; 19: 42–47.

44. Scheel O, Reiersen R, Hoel T. Treatment of tularemia with ciprofloxacin. *Eur J Clin Microbiol Infect Dis* 1992; 11: 447–448.

4

Food-borne zoonoses

Food-borne zoonoses are defined as 'those diseases contracted from eating foods of animal origin'. This is a broad definition and covers a wide spectrum of pathogens, although the most important on a day-to-day basis are mostly bacteria.

The importance to our society of food-borne zoonoses must not be underestimated. Our domestic system of agricultural production is regulated to reduce transmission of disease into the food chain, and considerable sums of money are expended annually to make our food safe. Retailers have a vast responsibility to handle food correctly and inspections should be carried out regularly by local and national enforcement bodies to ensure that the provisions of a wide range of regulations are complied with.

In the event of a profound failure in the system, by either an unforeseen emerging infection or a system or regulatory failure, the effects can be profound, for example, bovine spongiform encephalopathy (BSE) or the *Escherichia coli* outbreak at Wishaw, Scotland. It can be very difficult after such occurrences to deal with ensuing public fear or panic, whether justifiable or not. The media have been often vilified, with some justification, for escalating some dramas into crises.

This said, food safety, the protection of the public and addressing the concerns of consumers and their organisations are of paramount importance. The prevention of unnecessary disease, whether mildly inconvenient or fatal, has to be the concern of all individuals and organisations involved in food supply and public health and safety. Within the realm of healthcare professionals, those patients seen with infections acquired from food may have already been failed by some of the safety measures normally in place; although inability to store, handle or cook food correctly can also be a potential source of such infections.

Typical transmission pathway

An animal suffering from a disease, which may be inapparent, creates a product of either milk or body tissue in which the causative organism is entrained. This product is then either further processed or directly passed to a final consumer who then either with or without cooking eats the contaminated item and then in susceptible cases develops the disease after a variable incubation period.

Food-borne zoonoses associated with fish

The most significant disease sometimes associated with fish is cholera, although as humans are one of the main reservoirs for the disease there is a continuing debate as to its status as a zoonosis.

Of more potential significance is a complex of diseases associated with certain types of planktonic algae called dinoflagellates. These produce toxins which then accumulate in shellfish and certain other fish. Sporadic outbreaks may relate to weather, tidal, current and ambient temperature/sunlight.

The disease known as ciguatera is associated with farmed salmon and can also be caused by consumption of tropical and subtropical marine fish. This disease now occurs worldwide due to transportation of fish to geographically distant regions for the gourmet restaurant trade.[1]

Transmission occurs when contaminated fish is consumed. Symptoms commence with perioral numbness and tingling, which may become generalised. Nausea, vomiting and diarrhoea may follow as the condition progresses. Neurological symptoms include paraesthesia, arthralgia, myalgia, headache and acute temperature sensitivity. Vertigo and muscular weakness may also be seen.

Cardiovascular involvement with bradycardia, tachycardia and hypotension can occur.

The condition is usually self-limiting, and symptoms regress within several hours or days. In isolated cases neurological symptoms can persist, although normally there is no permanent damage.

In cases of poisoning following ingestion of shellfish a complex of afflictions is seen depending on the variety of toxins ingested. These vary depending on the different groups of dinoflagellates responsible. In general, saxitoxin derivatives cause paralytic shellfish poisoning (PSP), okadaic aid and yessotoxin cause diarrhoeic shellfish poisoning (DSP), brevetoxins cause neurotoxic shellfish poisoning (NSP), and domoic acid causes amnesic shellfish poisoning (ASP).[2]

In serious cases, if the individuals were to get all of the poisoning symptoms together, they would not be able to speak, they would be numb all over, the bottom would be dropping out of their world, and they would not know why.

The last publicised case of DSP in the UK occurred in June 1997. Forty-nine people ate mussels or mussel-containing soups at two London restaurants. These mussels originated in UK waters. It was the first incident in 30 years attributable to domestic shellfish. DSP toxins were first detected in shellfish from the Thames estuary in 1991: no previous outbreak had occurred in the UK. An incident in 1994 related to consumption of imported shellfish.

No cases of ASP have been reported in the UK. Where the disease does occur it is believed to be worst in elderly patients, and fatalities have occurred. The last case report of PSP in the UK was in 1968. This condition is particularly dramatic as the toxins can cause respiratory paralysis and, unless supportive therapy is given, death follows rapidly.

The Ministry of Agriculture, Fisheries, and Food (MAFF: now the Department for Environment, Food, and Rural Affairs (DEFRA)) has a system of location warnings geared towards preventing dinoflagellate-contaminated crustacea and fish being harvested from affected sea and tidal areas. The warnings are generated by analysis of shellfish harvested from monitoring sites at a number of indicator sites around estuaries and coastal waters.

Elsewhere in the world all of these diseases are significant, especially in tropical waters. Most international fish-trading nations have established similar monitoring systems.

Food-borne zoonoses associated with meat

Most of the UK population still eats meat, although vegetarianism is on the increase. Meat may be consumed as discrete cuts, comminuted meat products, i.e. beefburgers or sausages, processed items such as spam or corned beef, and cured, smoked or salted products. The exact source of any outbreak can be linked to dietary preference which is usually set by cultural factors and prevailing religious belief. This can protect or expose populations to a variable spectrum of pathogens. The bacteria within this next ection, however, form a universal threat to human health. The following section deals with probably the most serious pathogen of this group.

Escherichia coli

E. coli forms a part of most mammalian bacterial gut flora. It has a vast array of serotypes: some are benign, while others are dramatically pathogenic. This can vary from species to species; a benign form in one animal may be a deadly organism in another.[3]

The particular serotype of major concern is O157:H7, which was first identified as a major cause of serious outbreaks of food poisoning in the USA and Canada during the 1980s. This serotype is variously known as enterohaemorrhagic *Escherichia coli* (EHEC) or Vero cytotoxin-producing *Escherichia coli* (VTEC) O157. There are other serotypes which can produce similar clinical disease; however, this is both the most commonly seen in clinical cases and also the most severe. The Public Health Laboratory Service (PHLS) figures show approximately 1250 cases of *E. coli* O157 infection annually, of which approximately 50% are food-borne.[4]

Transmission

Disease in humans follows the consumption of food, usually meat or meat products, milk or water, which have become contaminated with faecal material. Direct contact with infected animal faeces has also been shown to be an efficient means of transmission. The organism is particularly associated with ruminant animals, especially cattle, sheep and goats. Current estimates from DEFRA, following an extensive survey across the whole of the UK of animals at slaughter, indicates that approximately 4.7% of cattle and 1.7% of sheep demonstrate asymptomatic faecal carriage of this serotype. Another survey carried out on live beef cattle in Scotland showed that 8% of animals shed the viable pathogen in their faeces.

Contamination of carcasses with faeces at slaughter has also been demonstrated. Meat from such carcasses poses a considerable risk if jointed, sold and subsequently consumed undercooked. To prevent or reduce infection from this source, recommendations have been made that vets at abattoirs assess the faecal load of the animal's body surface before slaughter. Any animals likely to produce carcasses with high levels of possible contamination should be rejected, further cleaned and resubmitted, or processed with particular attention to hygiene procedures and additional precautions, as deemed necessary. Contamination may also occur following contact between cooked products and raw meat, or the instruments or surfaces used whilst processing raw meat. The inoculum necessary to initiate progression to clinical disease has been estimated at fewer then 100 viable organisms.

Outbreaks may be sporadic, and may only affect single individuals; these are often associated with animal faecal contamination of water or milk. Collective outbreaks with large numbers of cases usually stem from breakdowns in controls within catering establishments. During a widespread outbreak, there may be secondary spread from patient to carer, or other person-to-person transmission.

Disease in humans

Once in the gastrointestinal tract the organism adheres to the gut wall where it proliferates and produces a toxin that is capable of damaging the gut lining to a variable degree. Only 30% of those who become infected show symptoms. The effect of the toxin may cause solely fluid loss and diarrhoea; in more severe cases there is also haemorrhage into the gut lumen and this is known as haemorrhagic colitis (HC). The condition can progress to haemolytic–uraemic syndrome (HUS), especially in children, with kidney damage that may progress to full renal failure with associated haemolytic anaemia and occasionally death. HUS occurs in roughly 5–10% of clinical cases. The organism is now recognised as the main cause of HUS in children. Recently there has been some evidence[5] that the development of HUS may be linked to the use of antibiotics in patients, with the drugs rapidly killing the bacteria, and producing massive toxin release. In adults (especially the elderly), but also occasionally infants, the course may be slightly different. Neurological disturbances may develop in addition to the HUS symptoms: this complex is known as thrombocytopenic purpura (TTP), and fatalities follow its development.[5]

Treatment

Treatment is supportive, as there is no specific treatment that shortens or ameliorates the course of the disease. Rehydration is essential; dialysis may be necessary, especially where there is significant kidney involvement. If kidney failure occurs, short-term dialysis followed by later kidney transplantation is the only option. As previously mentioned, the use of antibiotics is considered to be inappropriate.

Incidence

The incidence of infection is apparently on the increase, with 361 cases in the UK in 1991, compared to 1429 in 1999. However, this could reflect increased awareness and better screening techniques. The major risk groups affected are infants, children, elderly or immunocompromised individuals. There appears to be a seasonal pattern of infection – statistics show an increase in reporting during August and September. Within the

UK there is also a characteristic geographical spread, with more cases being reported in Scotland and northern England.

Anatomy of an outbreak

The chronology of the last serious outbreak of *E. coli* O157 poisoning in Scotland is shown in Table 4.1 to demonstrate how an outbreak can develop, and to highlight some of the issues related to controlling the spread of food-borne disease.[6]

Table 4.1 Anatomy of an outbreak: Wishaw timeline and statistics

17 November 1996	A pensioners' lunch is held at Wishaw Parish Church; the buffet is provided by J. Barr and Son, Butchers of Wishaw (initial infection)
22 November 1996	The possibility of outbreak of *Escherichia coli* O157 is identified after a history is taken from nine of 15 confirmed or suspected cases. Eight of the nine consumed food directly or indirectly from J. Barr of Wishaw
23 November 1996	A birthday party is held at the Cascade Public House in Wishaw, with J. Barr as caterer. Outbreak control team established
24 November 1996	Barr's product chain is properly identified and its full extent mapped. There was an extensive supply and distribution network with meat and meat products being supplied to 85 outlets in central Scotland
26 November 1996	The first food hazard warning is issued
27 November 1996	The Wishaw premises of J. Barr are closed down
15 December 1996	The last case of infection linked to products from this source is reported
20 January 1997	The outbreak is declared over

In any outbreak, it can be difficult to identify the focus. In this case, as in many epidemics, it was difficult to identify the problem until people became ill. History-taking becomes very important, as it is often the only key to identifying the source of the infection.

Once there was a presumption that an outbreak was occurring, an outbreak control team was formed which met daily during the outbreak until it was controlled. This allowed successful coordination of health service matters with local and regional government environmental health agencies. It also formed a forum for epidemiology and other specialist support to be discussed and implemented in forming policy and strategy to control the outbreak.

It is of great significance that J. Barr was not solely a butcher. His premises also had a bakery and purveyed raw meat, cooked meat products and bakery items, which were sold from the premises, and also distributed as wholesale goods over a wide geographical area. Although attempts had been made to improve the premises, cross-contamination of cooked products and raw meat was possible, and is thought to have led to the outbreak.

The records of the transactions involving sale and supply of products from the Wishaw premises were complex, and sometimes vague. It took a considerable amount of time and effort for health officials to ascertain their full extent. This allowed contaminated products to remain on sale for longer than was desirable. J. Barr and Son had more than 400 employees, including part-time workers, who lived in the local area, all of whom had to be tested, taking time and effort away from other areas.

For all of these reasons, this outbreak was serious and extensive. The lessons learned from this outbreak have informed later legislation and practice, with enhanced requirements for record-keeping and food hygiene.

Case statistics

Over the period of the outbreak, of 969 incidents of food poisoning reported, 496 were viewed as suspected cases. Of these cases, 272 were confirmed, 60 were classified as probable, and 164 as possibly linked.

A total of 127 people were admitted to hospital: 13 required dialysis and 18 died. Three further patients died later from complications associated with infection, giving a final figure of 21 fatalities for the outbreak. Of the dead, eight had attended the Wishaw Church luncheon, and six were residents of Bankview Nursing Home, to which cooked meats from J. Barr had been supplied. The 18 people who died during the outbreak were all over 69 years of age.

The fatal accident inquiry subsequent to the outbreak found that the fault lay with John Barr, and also the Environmental Health Department of the local council. Mr Barr was tried for recklessly supplying contaminated meat but acquitted and has since been privately sued for damages by about 120 people.

The significance of this outbreak cannot be underestimated. At the time this was the second-highest number of deaths associated with an *E. coli* O157 outbreak anywhere in the world. It was only surpassed by an outbreak in Japan in 1996 where nearly 10 000 people were infected, with an associated mortality in excess of 30 individuals.

There have been a number of later unrelated outbreaks of significance. In the Tayside outbreak on 31 January 1997, six elderly people in a nursing home were infected by food contamination, of whom three died. There was also an outbreak in Cumbria on 5 March 1999 linked to faulty pasteurisation. In the latter incident there were no fatalities. Following heavy rain and contamination of a scout camp in Banff, Scotland, 18 clinical cases were reported.

A number of sporadic cases have also occurred linked to contaminated water supplies or contact with raw sewage. Most cases have been seen in children: a 2-year-old girl died in Alvah, Banffshire, following ingestion of contaminated water in September 2000, and another girl became fatally ill after playing on Dawlish beach in Devon. Two other children also contracted the disease in the same outbreak, but both made full recoveries.

The Pennington report

Following the outbreak at Wishaw, Professor Sir Hugh Pennington was commissioned to investigate and make recommendations for future control of the disease. The group he chaired produced a report that made 32 recommendations. The main points were that there should be enforced separation of cooked and raw meat at catering premises, a programme of lessons on food handling for children and an *E. coli* awareness programme for farm workers. Additionally it was recommended that all butchers should be licensed, with one of the conditions of gaining and maintaining accreditation being mandatory staff training.[6]

The report's recommendations led to a media furore and, together with fears over *Listeria* and *Salmonella* and the onset of the BSE/variant Creutzfeldt–Jakob disease (vCJD), formed part of the demand for the establishment of a Food Standards Agency (FSA) in the UK.[7]

Listeriosis

Listeriosis is an often serious infection, caused by eating food contaminated with the bacterium *Listeria monocytogenes*. In the UK during 1998 there were only 110 clinically proven cases reported to the PHLS. This number shows a marked decline, which has occurred since guidance was issued in 1988 by the Chief Medical Officer (CMO). In the USA, despite health warnings from various responsible government agencies, an estimated average of 1850 persons become seriously ill with this disease annually, of whom in excess of 20% die. Refrigerated products can spread the disease, as *L. monocytogenes* is capable of slow growth at low temperatures.

Transmission

L. monocytogenes is found in soil and water. Vegetables can become contaminated from the soil or from manure used as fertiliser. Animals can carry the bacterium without appearing ill and can contaminate foods of animal origin, such as meats and dairy products. The bacterium has been found in a variety of raw foods, such as uncooked meats and vegetables, as well as in processed foods that become contaminated after processing, such as soft cheeses and cold cuts at the deli counter.

Unpasteurised (raw) milk or milk products made from unpasteurised milk may contain the bacterium. Humans and animals may also contract the disease by direct contact with infected faecal matter. A cutaneous form of the disease can occur from such contact. Transfer of the pathogen from mother to fetus or neonate has been well documented, as has infection following inhalation of infected aerosols, again in both humans and other animals. Venereal spread has been documented in cattle. It is estimated that 5% of the human population carries the bacterium asymptomatically in the gut.[8]

Risk groups

The main significant risk group is pregnant women. The disease can affect both mother and baby, and fetal or neonate death may follow maternal consumption of contaminated products. In an outbreak in North Carolina, USA, following the ingestion of infected soft cheese, of 11 women presenting with clinical signs, 10 were pregnant. As a result there were five stillbirths, three premature births and two infected neonates required treatment.[9]

Immunocompromised patients, from whatever cause, are also likely to suffer serious illness, with fatalities in serious cases. This is also true for the elderly or infirm patient. In otherwise healthy individuals, infection is possible; however, they are less prone to display serious or fatal sequelae. A study in the USA[10] has also established that patients who use quantities of antacids or who take cimetidine may be at increased risk of contracting disease, due to the inhibition of gastric acid. It is not known whether this also applies to patients receiving proton pump inhibitors.

Disease in humans

In most cases, infection occurs following ingestion of contaminated foodstuffs. There is a prepatent period of up to 10 weeks following infection. Clinical onset usually follows fever, headache, nausea and vomiting and symptoms similar to a severe chill. Abdominal cramps, stiffness of the neck and photophobia may also be present. The condition may progress with organ involvement, including endocarditis, internal lesions, metritis, septicaemia and meningitis. As central nervous system involvement becomes more widespread, there may be convulsions, confusion and vertigo.

Focal necrosis in the placenta may occur with spontaneous abortion, premature birth or infective transfer to the baby at birth. Babies may display a septicaemic infection within the first week after birth, or a septicaemic form with associated pneumonia within the first month of life.

A fatality rate of higher than 20% of clinical cases has been seen when treatment is not made, or is not commenced quickly.

Treatment

There is no vaccine available to prevent listeriosis in humans or animals. Treatment options are limited to the use of supportive measures and antibiotics.

Oral penicillins, especially amoxicillin at high doses by mouth, i.e. 500 mg three times daily for 5–7 days, have been shown to be effective. Erythromycin can be substituted in patients who are allergic to penicillin, at a dose of 500 mg four times daily for 1 week.

In serious cases, penicillin or ampicillin has been used successfully either intravenously or by mouth at high doses. Ampicillin plus gentamicin, or trimethoprim/sulfamethoxazole has also been used; however, this is normally reserved for secondary care usage under the control of expert opinion and monitoring. Even with prompt treatment some infections result in death. Use of recombinant DNA tests has been trialled to speed diagnosis and treatment.

Prevention

Listeria is killed by pasteurisation, and heating procedures used to prepare ready-to-eat processed meats should be sufficient to kill the bacterium; however, unless good manufacturing practices are followed, contamination can occur after processing.

The general guidelines recommended for the prevention of listeriosis are similar to those used to help prevent other food-borne illnesses, such as salmonellosis. Food from animal sources should be thoroughly cooked, especially beef, pork and poultry. Raw vegetables must be washed thoroughly in clean water before eating. Uncooked meats, vegetables and cooked or ready-to-eat foods should be stored separately or segregated. Unpasteurised milk or milk products should be avoided. General food hygiene precautions apply – knives, cutting boards and hands should be washed after each occasion of handling uncooked foods.

Recommendations for persons at high risk, such as pregnant women and persons with weakened immune systems, are in addition to the recommendations listed above. In 1988 the following advice was issued by the CMO:

> The CMO has established that the incidence of listeriosis in pregnancy stands at 1 in 30 000 live and stillbirths. Pregnant women should avoid certain ripened soft cheese, feta, Brie, Camembert, blue-veined cheeses such as Danish Blue, Stilton and Gorgonzola, and Mexican-style cheeses. Additionally they should not consume meat-based pâté. Cheddar and Cheshire-type cheeses, or soft fresh cheeses such as cottage cheese or fromage frais, do not pose a threat as they rarely contain *Listeria* or, if contaminated, carry insufficient organisms to cause infection. The same is true of processed cheeses, which have often undergone pasteurisation. Pregnant women should reheat chilled meals and ready-to-eat poultry thoroughly until piping hot. They should not assist with lambing, milk recently lambed ewes, touch the afterbirth or come into contact with newborn lambs. These recommendations also apply to immunodeficient individuals. Healthy children more than 4 weeks old are not at risk.

This advice is still current and valid.

Case histories

During January 2000, following two deaths in France, Coudray, producer of a variety of meat products, was forced to disinfect its factory completely. In 1992 the same factory was the source of a *Listeria* outbreak in which, of 279 cases, 63 people died and 20 women aborted their babies.[11]

The deaths of a 75-year-old man and a baby less than a month old were linked to consumption of pork-based coarse pâté by the pensioner and the mother of the baby. In February 2000 these deaths were followed by seven more, including two other infants.

Coudray exported widely within and without Europe, so an extensive product recall and publicity campaign was mounted to stimulate consumer awareness. In France, health authorities were unable to iden-tify the source of infection that left another 23 people ill across 19 regions of the country.

In August 2000, analysis of ice cream produced at a North Wales creamery was found to contain *Listeria*. Production was halted, and on investigation faulty processing was found to be to blame.

Salmonella

In 1988, in a statement made to the House of Commons, Edwina Currie (a then junior Health Minister) stated that 'most egg production is con-taminated with *Salmonella*'. The resulting media frenzy and reaction from the public forced her to resign from her post. An investigation was launched in response to her statement, and in 1989 a cull policy was introduced to try and control the incidence of the disease. Two million chickens were slaughtered – with no detectable effect on disease inci-dence. It is estimated that one in every 700 eggs laid today will be infected. The monitoring and testing for *Salmonella* and other food-borne pathogens was tightened after this débâcle.

On the basis of the outbreak data available from the PHLS it is believed that 90% of all *Salmonella* infections affecting humans are derived from food. In a major study of infectious intestinal disease (IID) carried out in England in 1994–1995, there were approximately 94 000 cases of *Salmonella* food poisoning.[4]

Salmonella enteritidis is the main culprit in fish and poultry. Other *Salmonella*, including *typhimurium, agora, montevideo* and *enteretia* (*paratyphi* spp.) are also clinically significant. *S. typhimurium* is primar-ily associated with cattle but has also spread to pigs, sheep and poultry. Certain of the 2300 serotypes appear to be particularly invasive, includ-ing *S. virchow* and *S. java*. Reported cases of *Salmonella* show a distinct consistent seasonal pattern, with a peak of infection observed in August.

Comminuted meat products and eggs have been identified as the main source of infection, especially sausages and burgers, although the microbes have also been found in beef, pork, chicken and, surprisingly, cereals. Some *Salmonella* spp. have been isolated from foodstuffs as diverse as spices, vegetables and fruit.

Disease in animals

Animals may be asymptomatic carriers of *Salmonella*. They may also suffer clinical disease with intestinal disturbance, septicaemia and death.

Spread within herds or flocks can be rapid, with disastrous results. *Salmonella* spp. are also an issue in companion animals. Dogs, cats and particularly reptiles can also act as carriers.

Transmission

Transmission usually follows ingestion of infected food, or direct or indirect contact with animal faecal material.

Disease in humans

Symptoms include sickness, diarrhoea, abdominal pain and fever. The infection can also be inapparent and present as unexpected overwhelming septicaemia. Susceptible groups include the usual individuals, with the elderly, very young, infirm and immunocompromised being at most risk. In the USA, recurrent *Salmonella* septicaemia is used as a marker for progress from human immunodeficiency virus (HIV)-positive status to acquired immunodeficiency syndrome (AIDS).

The most significant serotype in terms of mortality is *S. typhimurium* DT104, that shows 3% mortality. It is especially dangerous in the elderly. Infection with DT104 appears to be on the increase: there were 500 confirmed cases in the UK in 1991, rising by 1996 to 4000 (approximately 13% of total cases reported). There is also a threat from resistant serotypes, with 58% of *Salmonella* DT104 isolates being resistant to ampicillin, chloramphenicol, streptomycin, sulphonamides and tetracyclines. The R-serotype of this pathogen is additionally resistant to trimethoprim and quinolones.[12, 13]

Treatment

Treatment is usually symptomatic, using rehydration or antimotility agents such as loperamide. In severe or invasive cases ciprofloxacin or trimethoprim is used at doses related to the age and weight of the patient and the severity of disease.

Prevention

There is now statutory surveillance for all breeding flocks of poultry, and voluntary monitoring for all other flocks. A slaughter programme is in place, and any breeding flock found to be infected is isolated and culled. This ensures that chickens used for egg production commence their working lives free of *Salmonella* spp. Industry codes of practice have also been established to complement the statutory salmonella control programme. There is a vaccine available that can be used in laying flocks, and is used by many suppliers to the supermarket trade to ensure clean egg supply. These measures have resulted in a reduction in the number of human cases associated with poultry and eggs.

Animal feed is routinely tested for *Salmonella* and contaminated batches are rejected. Domestic precautions should be based on good hygiene practice in the kitchen, and ensuring food is adequately cleaned and cooked.

The British Egg Information Service has issued the following guidelines for consumers relating to the consumption of eggs: Consumers should avoid eating raw eggs; refrigerate unused or left-over egg-containing foods; discard cracked or dirty eggs; avoid cross-contamination of food by washing hands, cutting surfaces and plates after contact with uncooked eggs; and look for the lion logo and best-before date stamped on eggs. (The lion logo indicates that the eggs have been produced according to guidelines laid down by the Egg Marketing Inspectorate, a department of DEFRA with inspection and enforcement powers.)

Milk-borne diseases

Some of the zoonotic diseases that may be acquired from drinking infected milk will already be familiar from other chapters of this book. Brucellosis has been discussed in Chapter 3. There are still occasional cases of infection caused by *Brucella abortus*; however, *B. melitensis* has not been responsible for any cases of disease in the UK since case recording began. Surveillance for this organism is continually carried out by DEFRA.

Tuberculosis caused by *Mycobacterium bovis* needs no introduction. Human-to-human spread of resistant serotypes of *M. tuberculosis* is now more significant than the bovine form acquired from dairy products.

Q fever can also be spread by milk, and is deemed to be a serious zoonotic infection (see Chapter 3).

Mycobacterium avium subsp. *paratuberculosis* is found in raw milk and milk products. This organism is responsible for Johne's disease, a serious affliction of cattle worldwide. It can survive in soft cheese for up to 3 months and hard cheese for up to 10 months if the product is unpasteurised. In south-west England 1% of farms have cattle carrying the organism and an average of 2% of the herd is infected. It may be shed in the faeces of infected animals.

More heat-resistant than Q fever or tuberculosis, due to the clumping of its cells, it can survive pasteurisation. *M. paratuberculosis* has been suggested as one of several factors in causing Crohn's disease, although the evidence is conflicting.[14, 15]

The usual suspects

In addition to the previously mentioned organisms, cases of food poisoning may relate to a selection of the 'usual suspects'. They are all guilty as charged, and constitute a threat to consumers of badly or inadequately prepared food.

Clostridium spp. *perfringens, botulinum*

Clostridium perfringens, the causative anaerobic bacterium of many cases of gas gangrene, may also cause a food-borne disease. Widespread in the environment, and an inhabitant of the gastrointestinal tracts of humans and animals, it is often found in foodstuffs as a result of faecal contamination.

As with other forms of clostridial disease, it is the production of exotoxins by the pathogen that causes the main damage, especially where the ingested food carries a large inoculum, or heavy toxin load. The usual pattern of disease is linked to the ingestion of a number of viable *C. perfringens* that may produce clinical symptoms of abdominal cramps, diarrhoea and fever. The symptoms begin within 24 hours of ingestion and the clinical course is usually of short duration. Elderly patients and young children are most affected by this pathogen.

The more serious form, known as enteritis necroticans or pigbel, is linked to ingestion of a massive inoculum of *C. perfringens* type C. This form of the disease can be fatal, and is usually a result of inadequate cooking or slow cooling of cooked meats or meat products, with inadequate reheating, allowing the bacteria to multiply and produce quantities of exotoxin.

The clinical signs are linked to the effect of the exotoxin on the gut wall. Cell death and invasive necrosis lead to overwhelming septicaemia and circulating toxin levels that are toxic to major organs, including the heart, liver and kidneys (cf. gas gangrene). Diagnosis is often presumptive, confirmed by isolation of the organism or the exotoxin from a stool sample. Treatment is usually solely supportive.

Large outbreaks are usually associated with communal events or places and mass catering, either from professional or domestic sources, especially where food prepared in advance is not correctly stored. One of the largest thoroughly documented outbreaks occurred at a factory in Connecticut, USA. An employee banquet prepared for over 1300 people resulted in 600 cases, linked to previously prepared gravy, which had been incorrectly stored and inadequately reheated.[16]

Botulism

Botulism as a complex of disease states arises from contact with *C. botulinum* or its associated neurotoxin. As with other species of *Clostridium*, it forms spores which can survive desiccation and heat. It is often associated with ducks, geese and some other types of poultry. Cattle and horses have also been found to act as hosts for some strains. The organism is found in the environment, and also in the gastro-intestinal tract of infected mammals that may be asymptomatic carriers and amplifiers, although certain strains of botulism can affect them also.

There are no specific risk groups for botulism. It can affect anybody, anywhere at any time under the right circumstances. There are several distinct recognised types of botulism. These are food-borne, infant- and wound-associated. Luckily there is a very low incidence in the UK, with only a handful of cases annually.[17]

The food-borne form is not an infective form. It is solely caused by ingestion of botulinum toxin and is normally associated with products such as duck pâté, sausages and seafood, including smoked fish, which have been inadequately heat-treated, as the neurotoxin is destroyed at high temperatures. The amount of toxin necessary to cause clinical signs is measured in nanograms, thus, although foods ingested may contain no active bacteria, the residual toxin content can be sufficient to produce symptoms.

The disease usually begins 18–36 hours after the ingestion of the toxin. Early signs include gait difficulties, dysphagia and impaired vision. Respiratory distress, muscle weakness and abdominal distension and constipation may appear progressively. In severe cases assistance to maintain breathing by mechanical ventilation is required to prevent death. *Botulinum* antitoxin is used to treat the condition and, provided respiratory support is maintained, most cases will make a full recovery. The antitoxin may be obtained from locally designated centres throughout the UK, and in emergencies through the Department of Health Duty

Officer on telephone number +44 (0)20 7210 5371. There are cautions related to its use, as hypersensitivity reactions are not uncommon. Therapy should only commence after specialist advice has been obtained.

Many cases of food-borne botulism are believed to go undiagnosed, as the symptoms may be transient, and clinical signs may be confused with Guillain–Barré syndrome (see p. 150).

There was a single case of infant botulism in a child of 6 months in the UK during July 2001 that resulted in a recall of batches of formula baby milk. The disease stems from contamination of food with spores of *C. botulinum*, usually from environmental sources. There have only been six cases since 1978, and the last case was recorded in 1994. Confined to children under 1 year of age, the disease follows ingestion of viable spores. These become active, and over a period of days to weeks colonise the gut, producing the neurotoxin. This causes constipation and muscular weakness; the ability to control head movement is a particularly marked symptom, as well as a weak cry. There is marked lethargy, and a disinclination to feed.

As the loss of muscle tone and coordination progress, the child may become floppy, with respiratory distress. Diagnosis is made by isolating the organism from stool samples, or by toxin-testing faecal matter. Treatment with the antitoxin is not suitable, nor is antibiotic therapy, as this can cause massive death of the organism with overwhelming toxin release. Respiratory support may be necessary. Over time, even in severe cases, the paralysis lessens and there is usually a full recovery with no major sequelae.

One of the major food sources of *C. botulinum* is honey, and fears relating to infant botulism have led to advice that children under 1 year of age should not be fed honey. The gastrointestinal tracts of older children and adults have sufficiently robust bacterial flora to prevent the colonisation, even if active bacteria are ingested.

Wound-associated botulism is extremely rare, and follows the inoculation of an open wound with material containing either viable spores or active bacteria. The progressive production of toxins causes systemic paralysis radiating from the inoculation site. Treatment is usually with antibiotics, and antitoxin as necessary.

Yersinia enterocolitica

Of the same bacterial genus as plague, it is transmitted to humans by ingestion of foods as diverse as meat (pork, beef and lamb), oysters, fish and raw milk. It causes an acute-onset gastroenteritis with diarrhoea and vomiting, marked fever and abdominal pain. The pain can be so severe that it mimics appendicitis and has also led to misdiagnosis of Crohn's disease. It is capable of producing clinical complications that include septic arthritis, colonisation of existing wounds, bacteraemia and urinary tract infections. Luckily it is rarely fatal. The inoculum is usually traced to environmental sources, including soil and water; however squirrels, pigs and rodents form an animal reservoir.[18]

Cryptosporidiosis

Cryptosporidium spp. are spore-forming parasitic protozoans found widely in the environment in an extensive variety of foodstuffs, including salad and vegetables, raw meat and meat products, offal and milk, usually associated with contamination arising from animal faecal matter. *Cryptosporidium parvum* is considered to be a particularly significant pathogen. Calves, lambs and deer have been identified as asymptomatic animal reservoirs, capable of shedding viable organisms in their faeces.[19]

Transmission

Human infection follows either direct contact with animal faeces or consumption of inadequately cleaned or cooked products. There have also been recorded incidents of individuals contracting the disease after swimming in contaminated water. Person-to-person spread has been recorded, and is a particular risk in care settings.

Disease in humans

An inoculum of less than 100 encysted organisms can cause clinical disease. Following a prepatent period of between 2 and 14 days, and in individuals with no underlying risk factors, there is profuse self-limiting watery diarrhoea, with abdominal pain and cramps, and a low fever that may last up to 7 days. Loss of appetite and anorexia can follow with severe weight loss, especially in immunocompromised patients. There is also a high probability of relapse, with many patients having another bout of diarrhoea within 14 days of apparent cure.[20]

In patients with HIV/AIDS the disease may progress chronically, spreading to the bile duct, central nervous system and lungs. Unless treated swiftly, death will follow.

Treatment

In low-risk patients, treatment is purely supportive. Severe cases may need intensive care; however, treatment is difficult and as yet there is no specific therapy for conquering the pathogen. The strategy employed in HIV/AIDS patients centres on boosting the already damaged immune system with optimal retroviral therapy. There are some indications that those patients receiving clarithromycin or azithromycin with or without rifabutin for prophylaxis against *Mycobacterium avium* complex show less incidence of this disease.

Prevention

The pathogen can be destroyed by freezing, drying, heating materials to greater than 65°C, and irradiation. It is resistant to many disinfectants in common use.

Campylobacter spp.

Campylobacter is a much underrated cause of food poisoning. The pattern of infection in the UK is very different to the USA for this pathogen. In the UK, 80% of clinical cases are linked to contaminated food, whereas in the USA most cases are water-borne.

This particular pathogen is widespread and present in many farm animals. In particular, poultry is very susceptible to heavy bacterial loading. Under normal circumstances, the animals show no sign of disease, although there have been cases of abortion in sheep being linked to *C. jejuni*. The bacterium has been isolated from pigs, birds, cattle, dogs, cats, unpasteurised milk and water supplies. The measures in place to control *Salmonella* spp. have had little or no impact on the prevalence of *Campylobacter*. The two species considered significant in human disease are *C. jejuni* and *C. coli*, with the infective dose considered to be fewer than 100 viable organisms.

Transmission

The main route of infection is faecal contamination of carcasses ante- or postmortem.[21]

The organism is capable of surviving freezing and has been shown to survive for several months in frozen poultry and minced meat and also certain chilled foods. Thus cross-contamination could be a factor in infectious spread.

Disease in humans

The most immediate symptom of *Campylobacter* infection is a self-limiting diarrhoea of 2–10 days' duration, sometimes with bloody stools. *Campylobacter* mainly affects babies and young children, the immunocompromised and the debilitated. Other symptoms include fever, nausea and abdominal cramps that may vary from mild to severe, with occasional misdiagnosis as appendicitis, as with *Yersinia enterocolitica*. Symptoms may regress and reappear over a period of weeks. A septicaemic form has been seen in HIV/AIDS patients. Clinical cases of *Campylobacter* are associated with 20–40% of cases of Guillain–Barré syndrome. The triggering of reactive arthritis has also been associated with the disease. Following infection it is estimated that fewer than 1% of the population may become asymptomatic carriers.[22]

On average about 60 000 cases of *Campylobacter* infection are reported in the UK to the PHLS. During the IID study in England during 1993 to 1996 it was estimated that there were 870 cases per 100 000 head of population annually, with only one in eight cases being reported.

Treatment

In most cases the disease is controlled without resort to antibiotics. However, as it may be life-threatening in immunocompromised patients, antibiotics may have to be used.

Campylobacter displays high levels of resistance to fluoroquinolones, so any of the macrolide antibiotics are preferable; there are now some isolates which are dually resistant to both antimicrobial groups, which is a cause of some concern. In acute cases where resistance is suspected, tetracyclines, chloramphenicol and gentamicin have all been used. This is usually only initiated in secondary care settings after sensitivity testing has been done.

Prevention

The main control measure is the reduction of faecal contamination of carcass at and after slaughter. Hazard Analysis Critical Control Point (HACCP) measures, including keeping raw and cooked meats separate and ensuring that temperature-controlled processing of products is correctly undertaken, are effective in controlling spread through the food industry. In the home, using pasteurised milk and thoroughly cooking meat and poultry are recommended for everybody and especially for members of high-risk groups. Pets can carry and spread the organism and should be excluded from kitchens. The organism is sensitive to heat and drying, therefore thorough cooking acts as an effective control measure.

Guillain–Barré syndrome

Guillain–Barré syndrome can affect any individual, and is often associated with diarrhoea. It is an acute inflammatory episode in which demyelination of multiple neurons occurs. This can affect large portions of the peripheral neural network, and muscle weakness and paralysis may affect motor function, including breathing. Patients often require intensive care, especially if lung function is significantly impaired. Most patients recover, although convalescence may be prolonged. Luckily, fewer than 5% of cases are fatal. Some theories suggest that this may be an autoimmune disease triggered by bacterial or viral pathogens, of which *Campylobacter* is only one of several possible culprits. As yet there is no clear scientific evidence, although research is currently being undertaken.[23]

Food Standards Agency: scope and mission

In response to food scares, public concern over BSE, the Pennington report and a Department of Health study of the incidence of food poisoning in 1997, it was decided by government to set up a food standards agency.

The FSA is responsible for monitoring safety and standards of all food for human consumption, advising on diet and nutrition, and enforcing the law pertaining to food. It is also tasked with commissioning research into food safety. The Food Standards Act received royal assent in November 1999, and the appointment of Chairman Sir John Krebs was announced in February 2000. The FSA is directed by an executive board, appointed to act in the public interest, and is established so as not to represent particular sectors of industry or government. Its members come from a wide and varied background, and bring to their work a range of relevant skills and experience.

The stated aim of the agency is to 'protect public health from risks which may arise in connection with the consumption of food, and otherwise to protect the interests of consumers in relation to food'.

The FSA has initiated a campaign called 'from farm to fork', aimed at making food less contaminated and safer for the ultimate consumer. Initiatives have also been launched for clearer labelling, and to educate the public on food safety, nutrition and diet.

The FSA is accountable to Parliament through the Minister of Health. As a safeguard for its independence it has the unique distinction of being given by statute the legal power to publish the advice it gives to the government. The Meat Hygiene Service is now accountable to the Food Standards Agency.

Reducing zoonotic risks in food

Reducing the risks of zoonotic disease from foodstuffs is not just a process that begins and ends with the final consumer. Legislation and other physical measures to reduce or exclude pathogens from food are applicable to every step of the food chain, from field to table. Examining the process step by step will give some knowledge of the systems in place, and when considered against the information given in this chapter, allows some insight into the system failures that enable outbreaks to occur.

HACCP

One of the major food industry schemes for recognising and identifying risk and its remedies is the HACCP process. This is now internationally accepted as the preferred system for the management of food safety in food businesses. It has seven principles that provide a structured format for food safety by controlling hazards inherent in the food handling and production process (Table 4.2).[24]

Table 4.2 Hazard Analysis Critical Control Point (HACCP) principles.

HACCP is a systematic approach to the identification, evaluation and control of food safety hazards based on the following seven principles:
1 Conduct a hazard analysis
2 Determine the critical control points (CCPs)
3 Establish critical limits
4 Establish monitoring procedures
5 Establish corrective actions
6 Establish verification procedures
7 Establish record-keeping and documentation procedures

Food producers as well as government bodies, such as the Advisory Committee on the Microbiological Safety of Food, have endorsed it as the gold standard. The HACCP also applies to retailing and catering premises through current legal measures. The FSA has suggested that the principles should be extended to the agricultural process of food production, albeit in modified form. Until this is adopted widely, the current system of recommendation of a stepwise approach to infection control will continue.

General stepwise prevention strategies

Knowledge of zoonotic infections is the key to producing an effective stepwise programme. Understanding the likely routes of infection and the life cycle of the pathogen allows selective measures to be applied in a focused way, breaking the transmission route at its weakest point. The following generic points are used as an illustration only; a full case-by-case examination of all possible pathogens and their control is outside the scope of a book of this size. The references at the end of this chapter offer scope for deeper exploration of any or all of the topics raised.

Some of these measures may not be familiar or fully comprehensible to healthcare professionals. However, they do form a non-medical system for prevention of disease, and are no less valid than more therapeutically oriented methods.

Step 1: control the disease in the animal

The incidence of zoonotic disease in animals may be reduced by the use of vaccination, clean foodstuffs and water, and good housing and husbandry. Overcrowded or insanitary conditions can often lead to overt disease or unthrifty animals, requiring more therapeutic support for them to maintain sufficient health to attain slaughter weight or to continue to be productive. A reduction in infection rates has a dramatic effect on the incidence of infection further down the food or product chain. The associated lower levels of inoculum produce a lower likelihood of illness. The difficulties in implementing strategies at this point in the system are often economic – although the measures may be available, there may be little or no economic benefit to using them. Good housing and intensive staffing of livestock units are expensive, not only in capital outlay, but also in continuing infrastructure costs. In some cases those costs can become offset by higher prices for produce, but that is not always the case. The lobby for animal welfare and organic produce has improved the willingness of producers and consumers to follow this route, and it has been proven that there is a portion of the public who will willingly pay more for their food if it is of better quality. The converse is that there is also a need for food at the lowest price, and a bulk producer for a large supply contract may need to cut corners to stay in business, increasing perceived, if not actual risks.

Step 2: reduce contamination at harvesting

When eggs are picked out, or cows milked, the application of sensible hygiene precautions is essential. Eggs should be free of droppings and cleaned and date-marked. In dairies, the udder of the cow and the milking machinery should be as clean and hygienic as possible, with subsequent disinfection after each milking. Pipework and items such as clusters should be maintained and replaced as necessary to maintain adequate operating parameters. Milk should pass to the bulk tank and be subsequently chilled rapidly for later transport and pasteurisation.

At abattoirs, tight veterinary inspection both pre- and post-slaughter must be practised. Animals that display heavy faecal contamination should be cleaned or rejected. Slaughterhouse controls should prevent or reduce onward transmission into the food chain, with rejection of suspect carcasses. Prompt refrigeration of meat and careful cleaning of the carcass can reduce bacterial contamination drastically.

Step 3: retailing controls

Disinfection of working tools and areas, along with personal and premises hygiene procedures, protect consumers and workers from zoonotic infection. Sourcing products from assured suppliers, temperature and environmental monitoring and the separation of cooked and raw products reduce the possibility of amplification and transmission of infection. The tight control of 'use-by' and 'sell-by' dates is mandatory, as is periodic inspection by public health officials, and the implementation of monitoring of refrigeration and freezer plants.

Step 4: domestic precautions

In the home, consumers should use common-sense measures, including disinfection of surfaces and equipment, personal hygiene procedures and thorough appropriate cooking techniques. Using a refrigerator correctly and observing sell-by dates would prevent many cases of food poisoning.

It is perceived that the public in general has an acute need for education related to such matters, and the Health Education Authority and the FSA are to start a campaign aimed at addressing this problem.

General food hygiene recommendations

The FSA, the Food and Drinks Association and other public bodies have made various recommendations regarding food handling. These measures are designed to prevent cross-contamination of raw and cooked foods, and also to reduce the risk of consumers eating products that are raw or undercooked.

The advice is that people should clean surfaces, equipment and containers which have come into contact with raw meat. They must wash their hands after handling raw meat and before handling other utensils. The same plate should not be used for cooked and raw meat without washing the plate in between. Meat should be cooked until the juices run clear; this especially applies to burgers. Barbecues are considered to be particularly risky as meat may be not be fully cooked, and if previously chilled or frozen, may be raw or undercooked in the middle.

These recommendations were made after surveys had shown that public awareness of food hygiene was lamentable. Figures obtained from the Food and Drink Federation indicated that:

- 23% had never been taught to cook or prepare food
- 50% do not follow cooking instructions
- 15% admit not cooking meat fully or properly
- 25% do not always wash hands before cooking
- 10% do not separate raw meat from other foods
- 8% do not keep perishable items in a refrigerator

It appears from these figures that the general public has a profound need for education and information related to basic food safety and hygiene.

Miscellaneous items

Food sterilisation

Provision of appropriate information and an understanding of likely infections in risk groups form part of the support role of many hospital pharmacists. Knowledge of prevention strategies and animal handling guidelines is a valuable tool in the non-drug management of many patients.

Amongst the measures that may be needed in secondary care to manage the seriously ill patient is the non-technical issue of food provision. Sterilisation of foodstuffs, the education of food handlers and their screening as carriers of resistant organism serotypes may be necessary in certain care contexts, especially where immunocompromised patients are routinely treated.

Lower-input animals and higher-priced food

The continued debate over price as the sole arbiter of food supply, and the use of organic and high-welfare systems in agriculture, has a direct impact on zoonotic disease and antibiotic resistance. The use of older breeds of animal with lower input requirements in terms of therapeutic intervention and their higher innate resistance to infections, including zoonoses, is becoming increasingly important in agriculture.

This option for control of all zoonoses, and in particular those that are food-borne, will impact on the consumer. It will require considerable political will and willingness on the part of consumers to reach deeper into their pockets to make such initiatives commonplace.

The globalisation of food production and trading also has the potential to affect any country's domestic situation, and pathogens previously unknown in a country may be easily introduced on foodstuffs. There is still a debate raging over whether or not the epidemic of foot-and-mouth in the UK in 2000–2001 followed the importation of infected meat, which was fed in inadequately treated swill to pigs.

Farm visits

Recently there has been considerable adverse publicity surrounding cases of illness following farm visits, especially as there have been some fatalities in young children. Professor Sir Hugh Pennington, the eminent microbiologist who carried out the Wishaw inquiry and who has since advised government on zoonotic infection risks, has suggested that very young children should not visit farm premises because of the risk of infection.

The Health and Safety Executive has issued guidance to farmers under the Control of Substances Hazardous to Health (COSHH) provisions and there is a useful information sheet.[25]

Farmers must consider that visitors may also be exposed to contaminated faeces and other materials. Any farm open to the public should ensure that there are adequate washing facilities for visitors, with warm running water, soap and clean towels adjacent to all areas where the visitors may contact animals. Signs should be erected advising visitors to wash before eating, drinking or smoking, and also advising parents to check that their children do not put dirty hands or fingers in their mouths. Provision should be made for separate eating areas, close to washing facilities.

CASE STUDIES

Case study 5
Mr Kirkbride, a former Cameronian Highlander, has recently been treated for malignant melanoma, and has finished his chemotherapy with a good prognosis. He and his wife run a boarding kennel for dogs and cats. His wife comes in with a prescription for him. In addition to his normal medication he has been prescribed loperamide 2 mg capsules. When you take the completed script out to Mrs Kirkbride, she asks you about rehydration sachets, as his diarrhoea is profuse and watery. She expresses her concerns about the amount of weight Mr Kirkbride has lost since this problem had started; previously he had regained the several stone he had lost during his therapy. She says: 'He had even started to play with the dogs again and has been cleaning out their pens'.

Questions
1. Is Mr Kirkbride at risk?
2. If so, what are the likely causative agents?
3. What other risk groups might suffer from the same problem?
4. Suggest a management strategy for Mr Kirkbride.

Case study 6
A farmer's wife, Mrs McBride, comes into the pharmacy and purchases a pregnancy test. She returns a month later with a prescription for ferrous sulphate tablets and shows her maternity exemption certificate to your assistant.

You overhear her say to your assistant that at least she will be able to help with lambing before she becomes unable to work.

(continued overleaf)

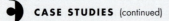

CASE STUDIES (continued)

Questions
1. Is it safe or desirable for Mrs McBride to help with lambing?
2. What are the risks, and the causative organisms?
3. What other activities related to agriculture should Mrs McBride avoid?
4. You know that the McBrides are famed for their unpasteurised ewe's milk matured soft cheese which they sell locally and nationally to the fine food trade. What advice should you give to Mrs McBride about preparing, working with or consuming these cheeses?

Case study 7
The local primary-school teacher seeks your advice. The headmaster of the school has proposed that the second-year children, aged 6–7 years old, should visit one of the local farms during lambing. The farm proposed is the property of one of the children's grandfathers, Mr Myers, and is a mixed-stock farm. The teacher wishes to know if it is safe for the children to go on this visit, and what facilities Mr Myers should be asked to provide when an arranged planning visit, prior to the class trip, takes place.

Questions
1. Should the visit take place?
2. What are the likely pathogens posing a risk?
3. What facilities should be in place on the farm for visitors?
4. What should parents try to stop their children doing to prevent disease problems on such a visit?

References

1. Swift A E, Swift T R. Ciguatera. *J Toxicol Clin Toxicol* 1993; 31: 1–29.
2. Todd E C D. Domic acid and amnesic shellfish poisoning: a review. *J Food Protn* 1993; 56: 69–83.
3. Tarr P I. *Escherichia coli* 0157:H7: clinical, diagnostic, and epidemiological aspects of human infection. *Clin Infect Dis* 1995; 20: 1–10.
4. Public Health Laboratory Service. *Statutory Notifications of Infectious Diseases; Notifications of Food Poisoning*. London: PHLS, 2001.
5. Wong C S, Jelacic S, Habeeb R L, *et al*. The risk of the hemolytic–uremic syndrome after antibiotic treatment of *Escherichia coli* 0157:H7 infections. *N Engl J Med* 2000; 342: 1930–1936.
6. The Pennington Group. *Report on the Circumstances Leading to the 1996 Outbreak of Infection with E. coli 0157 in Central Scotland, the Implications for Food Safety and the Lessons to be Learned*. Edinburgh: Scottish Office, 1998.

7. Advisory committee on the microbiological safety of food. *Report on Verocytotoxin-Producing* Escherichia coli. London: HMSO, 1995.

8. Lorber B. Listeriosis. *Clin Infect Dis* 1997; 24: 1–11.

9. Anonymous. Outbreak of listeriois associated with homemade Mexican style cheese. North Carolina October 2000. *MMWR* 2001; 50: 560–562.

10. Ho J L, Shands K N, Friedland G, *et al.* An outbreak of type 4b *Listeria monocytogenes* infection involving patients from eight Boston hospitals. *Arch Intern Med* 1986; 146: 520–524.

11. Dorozynski A. Seven die in French listeria outbreak. *BMJ* 2000; 320: 601.

12. Anonymous. Multidrug-resistant *Salmonella* serotype *enteritidis* infection associated with consumption of raw shell eggs – United States, 1994–1995. *MMWR* 1996; 45: 737–742.

13. Wall P G, Morgan D, Lamden K, *et al.* Transmission of multiresistant strains of *Salmonella typhimurium* from cattle to man. *Vet Rec* 1995; 136: 591–592.

14. Thompson D E. The role of mycobacteria in Crohn's disease. *J Med Microbiol* 1994; 41: 74–94.

15. Hermon-Taylor J, Barnes N, Clarke C, Finlayson C. *Mycobacterium paratuberculosis* cervical lymphadenitis followed five years later by terminal ileitis similar to Crohn's disease. *BMJ* 1998; 316: 449–453.

16. Anonymous. *Clostridium perfringens* gastroenteritis associated with corned beef served at St Patrick's day meals – Ohio and Virginia, 1993. *MMWR* 1994; 43: 137–138, 143–144.

17. BBC News Online. Baby milk in botulism scare. http://news.bbc.co.uk (18 August 2001.)

18. Lindsay J. Chronic sequelae of foodborne disease. *Emerg Infect Dis* 1997; 3: 443–452.

19. Current W L, Garcia L S. Cryptosporidiosis. *Clin Microbiol Rev* 1991; 4: 325–358.

20. Fayer R, Ungar B L P. *Cryptosporidium* spp. and cryptosporidiosis. *Microbiol Rev* 1986; 50: 458–483.

21. Peterson M C. Clinical aspects of *Campylobacter jejuni* infections in adults. *West J Med* 1994; 161: 148–152.

22. Molina J M, Casin I, Hausfater P, *et al. Campylobacter* infections in HIV-infected patients: clinical and bacteriological features. *AIDS* 1995; 9: 881–885.

23. Bolton C F. The changing concepts of Guillain–Barré syndrome. *N Engl J Med* 1995; 333: 1415–1417.

24. Notermans S, Gallhoff G, Zwietering M H, Mead G C. The HACCP concept: specification of criteria using quantitative risk assessment. *Food Microbiol* 1995; 12: 81–90.

25. Health and Safety Executive. *Avoiding Ill Health at Open Farms: Advice to Farmers (with Teachers' Supplement).* AIS 23. Sudbury, Suffolk: Health and Safety Executive, 2000.

5

Variant CJD, BSE and other prion disease

For centuries sheep and goats have suffered from what had been a condition of unknown aetiology called scrapie. All attempts to identify or classify the causative agent had failed, although infectivity had been demonstrated by using an inoculum of brain tissue from sheep to sheep in the late 1930s. There has never been any demonstrable transfer of the causative agent of scrapie directly to humans and no associated clinical disease.

Until the last decade of the 20th century a 'slow virus' was suggested as the most likely cause, although no viral particle was ever isolated. The causative agent was known to be resistant to almost all methods and materials known to destroy or inactivate viral particles. Research workers in the 1990s identified a protein fragment which was apparently responsible for the affliction. These fragments were designated prions, and defined as 'small proteinaceous infectious particles which resist inactivation by procedures that modify nucleic acids'. The majority of scientists favour the prion theory: there is still some debate, and bacterial infections and manganese levels have been suggested as causative or additive factors in some bovine spongiform encephalopathy (BSE) or variant Creutzfeldt–Jakob disease (vCJD) cases.

The prion theory suggests that the responsible agent derives from protease-sensitive protein, a normal constituent of the cell membrane. Following a spontaneous or acquired genetic modification, this protein changes conformation so that it becomes protease-resistant. This change triggers a chain reaction: the rate of protein conformation change becomes exponential so that there is a rapid laying-down of the mutated form of protein (designated PrPsc – the sc for scrapie, the oldest known prion disease).

Prions are unconventional as an infectious agent. They consist of protein alone, with no nucleic acid. The diseases they cause are also different to any other infection or disease, as the evidence in all species shows that both infective material and hereditary factors have to be present for disease to occur.

The physical symptoms of the disease spectrum caused by prion agents arise from the alteration of cell-wall proteins into insoluble forms following exposure and incorporation of prion proteins. The process then becomes a self-sustaining chain reaction, which produces sheets of insoluble protein in neural tissue and particularly in the central nervous system, with inevitably fatal results.

It is now believed that, following infection by sufficient inoculum of aggressive prions, genetically susceptible individuals can develop the clinical signs of transmissible spongiform encephalopathies (TSEs) which affect most mammalian species. Their name reflects the finding on autopsy of brain and central nervous tissue riddled with holes like a sponge.

In 1997 Professor Stanley Prusiner won the Nobel Prize for Medicine for his discovery of prions (proteinaceous infectious particles), which contain no DNA or RNA. He postulates that prions may play a part in Alzheimer's disease, Parkinson's disease and other degenerative neural diseases.[1]

Animal TSEs

The best-known animal TSEs are bovine spongiform encephalopathy (BSE) affecting cattle, chronic wasting disease (CWD), which affects elk in northern America, scrapie affecting sheep worldwide with the exception of the Antipodes, and transmissible mink encephalopathy (TME) which affects mink, polecats and ferrets. There are also related feline/canine diseases and certain rodent diseases. It is difficult to substantiate some of these diseases in other species as they tend to appear slowly and are usually seen in the mature animal. For some species, attaining sufficient age to display the disease may not be achievable, as death from other causes intervenes before clinical signs are seen, and postmortem examination will not be possible or routine.

The two most significant TSEs in the UK at present are BSE and scrapie, which have an associated link to vCJD in humans. Although at the time of writing this linkage has not been conclusively scientifically proved according to some experts, the body of knowledge has reached a level of coincidence and circumstantial evidence that has the majority of the academic and lay population convinced.

BSE is a fatal neurological disease of cattle that was first identified in the UK in November 1986. The feeding of meat and bone meal (MBM) to cattle is blamed for its appearance in the national herd and this hypothesis had achieved wide acceptance by the end of 1988.

Changes in the way that animal carcasses were rendered before inclusion in the MBM appear to have enabled the prion agent to survive. The particular batch of MBM believed to be responsible for the outbreak probably contained material from sheep carcasses infected with scrapie, and particularly brain and spinal tissue. As little as 1 g of infected material in the feed is known to be able to cause BSE in 70% of those animals genetically susceptible to the disease. After clinical onset is observed the disease is rapidly fatal, within either a few weeks or months.[2]

By October 1996, BSE had been reported from 10 countries outside the UK. Some countries in western Europe reported cases in their native herds, probably arising from the importation of contaminated feed. Where other cases occurred they were unrelated to imported feed; however, these countries had imported livestock from the UK for breed improvement or other purposes. As it is now known that, once in the cattle herd, BSE can spread by maternal transfer; other cases arose in herds by this method. The only answer has been to undertake a slaughter policy to eradicate the disease.

A ban was put in place in July 1988 by the UK to prevent the inclusion of ruminant-derived protein in cattle feed. In November 1989 a voluntary ban supported by animal feed manufacturers stopped the inclusion of MBM in ruminant feeds. In 1990 this became law. Offal and other specified material became forbidden as an ingredient in animal feedstuffs under the regulations.

After the first appearance and identification of BSE in cattle, a dramatic rise in incidence was seen, some of which could have been solely attributable to better surveillance. Between 1987 and December 2000 more than 100 000 head of cattle identified as suffering from the disease were slaughtered. The numbers have declined dramatically from a peak in 1992–1993 of more than 30 000 cases a year to just over 1500 confirmed cases in the year 2000 (Figure 5.1). The guidelines that have been put in place to prevent recurrence and transmission into the food chain by feeding animal tissue to ruminants have been rigidly enforced and seem to be playing their part. Measures at slaughter to remove specified bovine material (SBM) from all cattle carcasses, and the strict inspection of meat at abattoirs, are aimed at preventing contaminated material from entering the food chain. SBM includes the head, spinal cord, tonsils, spleen, intestines and thymus gland. All SBM must be rendered (temperature-treated by boiling or steam-heating), and then destroyed. The material must not under any circumstances be included in material for human consumption.[3]

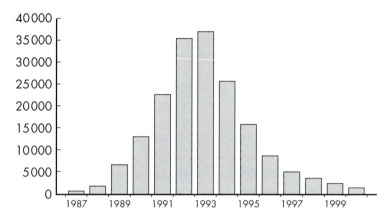

Figure 5.1 Confirmed cases of bovine spongiform encephalopathy (BSE) in the UK by year. Figures courtesy of the Department for Environment, Food, and Rural Affairs: http://www.defra.gov.uk/animalh/bse/index.htm.

Scrapie infection is important in our understanding of TSEs as it has been identified for the longest period, and before BSE appeared much work had already been done in trying to understand the disease and map its progress through the national sheep herd.

During this work it was realised how much an individual needed to be genetically susceptible to develop the disease. In research carried out in the 1950s a very dramatic study was undertaken. In the study, the same area of grazing already suspected to be contaminated with the infective agent (at that time not yet identified) was undertaken at the same time by two groups of sheep. The one was known to come from a scrapie-susceptible strain, the other from a genetic stock in which no clinical cases had ever been seen. In the first group all the sheep died having developed the clinical signs and symptoms, while in the second group none of the sheep died.

It is now known that in sheep, inoculation stems from grazing on pasture contaminated with placental matter or other bodily material. It is necessary for there to be both genetic susceptibility and the presence of infective agent for disease to occur. Once into a susceptible animal population, further spread can occur by maternal transfer, so that it becomes a genetic inherited disorder in future generations.

An infected animal can remain asymptomatic for a variable period of time. Clinical findings of scrapie in sheep are linked to the laying-down of prion protein cellular (PrPc) or PrPsc (scrapie) in infected cells. This is resistant to normal proteases, leading to sheets of protein forming in affected structures and their gradual infiltration with internal divisions, giving rise to segmentation and gradual, progressive destruction.

Certain sheep genotypes appear to be more susceptible to developing scrapie. Those sheep showing the Ala136Ala, Arg154Arg, Glu171Glu and Val 136 Val, Arg 154 Arg, Glu171Glu sequences in their genotype are known to be susceptible. Only one case of scrapie has been found in a sheep with Ala136Ala, Arg154Arg, Arg171Arg. There is no evidence of the prion responsible for scrapie being able to cross the species barrier directly into humans. Prion strain typing has shown scrapie to be closely related to the prion responsible for BSE in cattle, and that the causative agent of vCJD in humans is very close to BSE in its characteristics.

Human TSEs

At this point a digression is needed to examine what is known of TSEs affecting humans other than vCJD.

Creutzfeldt–Jakob disease

H.G. Creutzfeldt first described the disease now known as sporadic or classic Creutzfeldt–Jakob disease (CJD) in 1920. In 1921 another German neurologist, Jakob, described four more cases.

CJD appears to occur as a sporadic disorder in 90% of known cases. Most of the remaining 10% show a strong relation to a dominant inherited genetic trait. This was unexplained until the mapping of the human genome discovered that a mutation of chromosome 20 could lead to the damage necessary to initiate CJD. It appears that the genetic mutation, in association with ageing, produces a disease clinically indistinguishable from prion-mediated disease.

Several cases of CJD were related to the use of either brain tissue grafts originating from sufferers, or human growth hormone originating from the pituitary glands of cadavers. A case arose in 1974 following a corneal graft, and contaminated neurosurgical instruments have been implicated in several other cases. Following these cases a policy on destruction of surgical instruments and the use of synthetic hormones has prevented recurrence.[4]

The disease is invariably fatal and patients usually display a rapidly progressing state of dementia, with muscle spasm and tremor and a characteristic electroencephalogram (EEG) pattern. On autopsy, spongiform changes are found in the central nervous system.

The affliction occurs worldwide at a rate of about one case per million per year. There are higher rates in Slovakia and in a discrete group of Israelis who are all Libyan-born. In these groups one case per year per 10 000 is seen. This is attributable to the genetic mutation of chromosome 20 and the associated PrPc. CJD does not appear to be transmissible except genetically and there is no increase in occurrence in the partners of sufferers, nor is there any link to increased incidence in countries where scrapie is endemic.

A blanket study of cell samples from autopsy of large cohorts of cadavers has shown that as many as 1 in 10 000 people show signs of the mutation which can lead to CJD. It has also been suggested that, due to the limitations of the technique and the survey, this could be a substantial underestimate of the true incidence. Epidemiological surveillance of CJD was reinstated in the UK in 1990 to identify any changes in the occurrence of this disease after the epidemic of BSE in cattle.

Another human disease that appears to be related to similar but distinct genetic modifications, with slightly different clinical signs, is Gerstmann–Sträussler–Schenker (GSS) syndrome, first described in 1928–1936. This disease also appears to be familial, occurring in persons with an apparently hereditary predisposition, and a similar but different modification to chromosome 20. The rate of incidence of GSS is believed to be 2% of the rate of CJD, giving a case incidence of only 1 in 50 million per year.

The third of this quartet of human diseases is fatal familial insomnia (FFI), which was described in 1986 and seems to be similar in origin to CJD and GSS: it is related to an inherited genetic modification. Clinical symptoms begin with protracted untreatable insomnia and a gradual loss of coordination and motor ability. This leads to an increasing dementia. Sufferers cannot tell the difference between dreams and reality. Death occurs from 7–25 months after clinical signs of the disease appear.

The last of this group of diseases in humans is known as kuru. This disease state only exists in a single tribe from Papua New Guinea, the Fore Highlanders. A degenerative neural disorder, it was first described in 1957 by an Australian anthropologist. The disease was linked to the cannibalistic practice of eating deceased relatives' brains as part of an animistic religious rite. Since this practice has been discontinued the disease has virtually disappeared. Yet again the disease was characterised by gradual loss of neural capability. Postmortem findings of spongiform changes in the brain were also characteristic.

Our knowledge of kuru and scrapie, the identification of their method of spread, and how the disease progresses have been extremely important in gaining some understanding of the mechanism of spread of BSE and vCJD.

Variant Creutzfeldt–Jakob disease (vCJD) and BSE

Dr Robert Will first described vCJD in a 1996 paper in *The Lancet*. He stated: 'In the past few weeks we believe we may have identified a new clinico-pathological phenotype of CJD which may be unique to the UK. This raises the possibility of a causative link between BSE and CJD. The identification of a form of CJD that might be causally linked to BSE will result in widespread anxiety and concern'. This was an amazingly studied understatement.[5]

Initially known as new variant CJD, the 'new' designation for the disease was dropped by the Spongiform Encephalopathy Advisory Committee (SEAC) in March 1999, leaving the disease to be designated variant CJD.

The identification of this variant arose from a series of deaths and postmortem findings which, although having many of the characteristics of classic CJD, did not fit the accepted case profiles. When compared with classic CJD cases they were found to have an earlier age of onset, with a much longer period from clinical manifestation to death. The patients also did not have the characteristic EEG findings of sporadic CJD. At the time of the article in *The Lancet*, no similar cases had been seen in any other European country, thus triggering the possible link with BSE.

Patients suffering from vCJD had an average duration of illness of 2 years rather than the classic CJD pattern where it was unusual for a patient to survive for longer than 12 months. Classic (or sporadic) CJD affected patients aged 50–75 whereas vCJD affects a much younger group, with victims so far aged between 18 and 41 years.

Initially the hypothesis that vCJD and BSE were linked emerged from the association of two diseases of similar aetiology and clinical progress occupying the same location and time frame. It is now widely accepted that this disease is linked to BSE and that consumption of infected meat or other bovine material provides the inoculum (Figure 5.2). The evidence from studies in mice and monkeys supports the hypothesis.

It is still unclear how the prion invades the body after ingestion of infected material; however, a theory relating to Peyer's patches in the

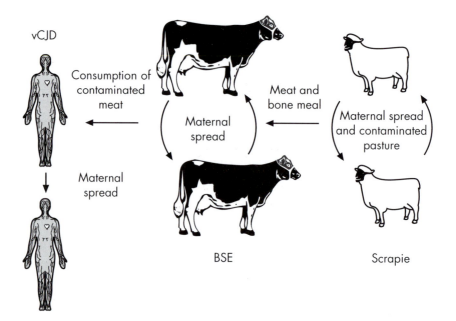

Figure 5.2 Diagrammatic representation of the most likely scenario for the emergence of variant Creutzfeldt–Jakob disease (vCJD). BSE, bovine spongiform encephalopathy.

gastrointestinal tract of children and young adults is currently under development. Peyer's patches allow pathogens to be presented to the immune system in a controlled manner so that immunity can be developed. They recede in size and number as the child matures into adulthood. The theory proposes that the prion is absorbed from the gut, ingested by mobile lymphoid cells and then travels to other parts of the lymph node system where it is subsequently able to develop in susceptible individuals. Neural pathways from the nodes can lead directly to the central nervous system, so the prion gains access by this route.

The cumulative number of definite and probable cases to 2 March 2001 totalled 95, including nine where no diagnostic confirmation will ever be possible as the bodies were cremated, or the relatives refused permission for exhumation and autopsy (Figure 5.3). The influence of genetic factors is demonstrated by the identification of a particular genetic variant in all of the cases tested to date. The associated variation of gene 20 has been found to occur in approximately 40% of the population of the UK. This does not exclude the possibility of people without this genotype of becoming victims of the disease.

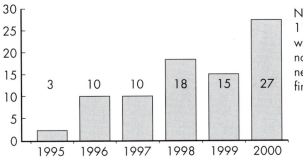

Figure 5.3 Number of deaths from variant Creutzfeldt–Jakob disease (vCJD) reported by year. Figures courtesy of vCJD Surveillance Unit.

In September 2000, the first report of possible maternal transmission of vCJD appeared. A baby born to a mother who subsequently died of vCJD was suspected of having the disease. The baby showed signs of brain damage with fits and convulsions, and was not developing normally. Confirmation of the diagnosis has not been possible to date; however, the possibility of such an event is consistent with the findings in both BSE and scrapie.

Disease symptoms

Victims initially present with non-specific psychiatric symptoms. The clinical disease presentation shows progression from anxiety, depression, to gradually worsening changes in behaviour.[6] Altered perception and painful sensory distortion are also seen in approximately 50% of patients.[7] There is a gradual loss of neuron density and function. After weeks, or months, the disease affects coordination and patients may have difficulty walking and picking things up; involuntary movements and convulsions occur. Memory problems develop and patients have reality perception difficulties, loss of motor control, dementia, paralysis and wasting. Patients deteriorate rapidly and require intensive nursing, as in the final phase of the disease total immobility occurs and the patient becomes mute. Death following overwhelming pneumonia is not uncommon.[8]

Diagnosis

Diagnosis in the initial stages of clinical onset is made difficult by the resemblance between this and other neurological and psychiatric disorders. Differential diagnosis relies on the use of magnetic resonance imaging (MRI), computerised tomography (CT) scans (Plate 6) and EEG. MRI scans have shown abnormal features in areas at the base of the brain in some vCJD patients, but the significance of these findings is not yet known. CT scans exclude other conditions, but do not definitively support the diagnosis. The use of lumbar puncture has proved of no benefit.[9]

The EEG findings in vCJD are consistently abnormal and do not show the distinctive changes associated with classic CJD. A mild elevation of hepatic enzyme levels has been seen, but is believed to be transient.

Confirmation of diagnosis is usually obtained only on autopsy, where the characteristic spongiform changes with microscopic findings of abnormal protein clusters encircled by holes are seen, resulting in a daisy-like appearance described as 'florid plaques'. A biopsy specimen has been obtained in some cases before death, which can confirm the diagnosis, but the process may distress both the patient and relatives so it is unlikely to be used routinely in the future. There are some indications that testing tissue from the tonsils may allow definitive diagnosis to be made without the need for invasive techniques.

A new test for CJD and related conditions has been trailed in the press during June 2001, although it is unclear when and if this will reach the stage of being a commercial reality.

Treatment for vCJD patients and the BSE inquiry

As has been previously stated, many patients suffering from vCJD are never properly diagnosed until after their demise. The disease is invariably fatal, and it is likely that by the time signs and symptoms are seen, and a presumptive diagnosis made, the disease will be well advanced and death will follow swiftly. As the disease presents in a dramatic way, with mental illness, anorexia and loss of motor function, there is considerable distress for both patient and relatives. Following the BSE report released by the government in 2000, decisions have been made to treat sufferers and their relatives in a more compassionate manner with coordinated action between agencies. A compensation scheme is also under development for victims and their families.[10]

In the interests of scientific research and public health, all patients suspected of suffering from a TSE are reported to the national Creutzfeldt–Jakob Disease Surveillance Unit (CJDSU), based in Edinburgh. Doctors from the unit visit all people with the disease and attempts are made to take a detailed history from the patient and relatives. The diagnosis of the case will also be reviewed at the same time. The CJDSU has produced a set of diagnostic guidelines which help place patients within classification groups of TSEs. Patients may be reclassified as their clinical symptoms and test results develop. Case notes are only closed after the death of the patient and when no further data are likely to be forthcoming.

The task of the CJDSU is to identify and investigate all cases of CJD and other TSEs in humans occurring in the UK. The unit is also responsible for a comprehensive national surveillance programme. The programme aims to track case trends over time, and to detect case clusters. Research is also being undertaken to detect risk factors and mechanisms of transmission. This work is aimed at determining the magnitude of the public health problem, and to produce informed prevention strategies and valid diagnostic tests.

The annual report of the CJDSU and its database work have allowed identification of two clusters of cases; these are examined extensively later in this chapter.

Treatment

Drug therapies have been tried in an effort to slow the progression of the disease. Amantidine and amphotericin, although effective at slowing or arresting the condition *in vitro,* have little or no effect on the disease in sufferers. Aciclovir, interferon, antibiotics, steroids and other antiviral agents have also been tried and have failed to alter the outcome significantly.

As patients deteriorate, rehydration and liquid feeds need to be used. Pain control may also be necessary. Clonazepam or sodium valproate can be given to control spasm and spasticity at normal doses, with titration to response. Sulphated glycosaminoglycans and Congo red are also proposed as possible starting points for therapies as they are both believed to affect PrP metabolism. Vidarabine is also currently under evaluation.

Future hopes for therapies centre around protein stabilisers to prevent conversion of normal protein into prion protein. Antigene therapies are also proposed: such agents would destroy the gene responsible for producing the prion protein; however, it is unclear if this modification would carry with it a risk that the responsible gene has other metabolic functions, which may be currently unknown, within normal healthy body systems. Even these therapies may only slow progression, and are not seen as effecting a cure.

During the late summer of 2001, there have been several announcements relating to the development of drugs and therapies that appear to offer some hope of slowing the progress of the disease. These have been welcomed by experts such as Professor Prusiner, and Dr Will of the CJDSU.

The BSE inquiry

The UK government set up the BSE inquiry in December 1997. The stated aim of the inquiry, led by Lord Phillips of Worth Matravers, Master of the Rolls, supported by Mrs June Bridgeman CB and Professor Malcolm Ferguson-Smith FRS, was:[2]

> To establish and review the history of the emergence and identification of BSE and new variant CJD in the United Kingdom, and of the action taken in response to it up to 20 March 1996. To reach conclusions on the adequacy of that response, taking into account the state of knowledge at the time; and to report on these matters by 31 December 1998 to the Minister of Agriculture, Fisheries and Food, the Secretary of State for Health and the Secretaries of State for Scotland, Wales and Northern Ireland.

As often happens in these affairs, the time frame became elastic. The report was finally received by the government in October 2000. It was published by the end of October and the then Minister of Agriculture, Nick Brown, welcomed its findings.

Patient issues

The inquiry found that standards of care and support for families varied widely and suggested that improvements were needed, including speedy diagnosis with informed, sympathetic advice to relatives about the future course of the disease and the needs of the patient. It is now recognised that there is a requirement for rapid assistance for families to allow victims to be cared for in their own homes and access to hospice or similar care settings in the final phases of the disease's progress.

The necessary measures include many of the items of care normally seen in association with care for the elderly, disabled or cancer sufferers. They include home adaptations, respite care and, especially if the victim is the main breadwinner, monetary support.

Because the average age of the victims so far has been low in comparison to classic CJD, specialist strategies were not previously in place for dealing with young victims of degenerative disorders. Another proposal made in response to the report's findings has been the provision of beds in hospices or other facilities for the terminal care of sufferers. Much of the healthcare professional input in the care of victims of vCJD is palliative and relies heavily on good nursing practice. It has been found that many staff have become distressed and shocked whilst carrying out their duties in support of patients and their relatives due to the nature and rapidity of the disease's progress.

The problem of vCJD/BSE in the UK crosses many of the boundaries between government departments. The Ministries of Agriculture, Health and Social Services have, for once, agreed a package of measures to support the victims and their families.

The Department of Health has also decided that, in future, a key coordinating worker will be appointed as soon as possible after diagnosis for every patient. The key worker will be responsible for ensuring that there is an adequate care package in place, not only for the sufferer but also for relatives. The national care coordinator for vCJD treatment is currently the CJDSU.

In the event of a rapid rise in the number of cases, the government and the Ministries will review the arrangements for a care fund and may alter arrangements so that they operate on a regional rather than the current national basis.

Epidemiological clusters

Through the work of the CJDSU, two clusters of cases have been identified. The inquiries carried out by the local health authority in the Leicestershire cluster have produced interesting insights into how the disease is contracted.

The Leicestershire cluster

A cluster of cases of vCJD was first identified in the Leicestershire village of Queniborough in November 1998. In July 2000, when the investigation began, the number of possibly linked cases had risen to five. Between August 1996 and January 1999 five people developed the disease and subsequently died. All the victims lived in the area between 1980 and 1991, and therefore the investigation concentrated on this period as this was the only time period when a common exposure could have occurred.

Clusters of cases form a very important part of the tools available to epidemiologists to identify not only past exposure and infection pathways, but also future trends. Following an investigation the expert findings were released in March 2001. At the outset of the investigation a number of risk factors were excluded as linking the victims. These included surgery and blood transfusions, dental surgery, occupational exposure, immunisations, injections, body piercing, cuts and animal bites, baby foods, school meals, drinking water and high manganese levels. All of these factors had been postulated as causing or contributing to the development of vCJD, and are either under investigation or have been identified as non-contributory factors.

Scope of the investigation   The investigation encompassed the farming practice prevalent in the late 1980s when BSE was first identified in cattle. At that time local beef cattle were raised alongside dairy cattle and were therefore fed meat and bone meal (MBM) from the age of 6 days rather than 6 months. They therefore had a greater lifetime exposure to the BSE agent in meat and bone meal than normal beef cattle.

In this area there was a moderately high number of cases of BSE on farms that supplied fattened cattle for beef, and therefore it was reasonable to suppose that some of the meat could come from infected beasts. The beasts supplied for meat were unusual, as they were Friesian–Hereford crosses derived from the dairy industry. Such animals are slow to fatten and were therefore slaughtered at 30–36 months of age, rather than at the younger age normally associated with beef breeds. Being older, and given their feeding pattern, it was more likely that these animals could have had subclinical BSE at slaughter. Therefore it was more likely that their meat was infectious.

Slaughter and butchery practice   The investigation found that most butchers in the area, as with most others nationally, bought their meat in from wholesale suppliers who bought from a variety of slaughterhouses. These slaughterhouses selected beasts from a wide variety of cattle markets and auctions across an extensive geographical area. A minority of butchers selected their own beasts at the local cattle market, and would then subsequently slaughter them themselves or have them processed at a nearby abattoir.

The investigation also covered slaughtering practice of large and small abattoirs in the area from the early 1980s. Cattle were slaughtered using a captive bolt as usual; however, in some local abattoirs and butchers, a pithing rod was also used to prevent the beast kicking after slaughter. The use of a pithing rod ruptures the brain structure and is more likely to release infective material into the work area, or onto the carcass, especially as the prion is most concentrated in brain material. Some local butchers also removed the brain from the head of the beast for further processing, increasing the chance of contaminating the meat.

Small abattoirs also often used a cloth to wipe down the beast after slaughter to remove any unwanted tissue, rather than hosing the carcass down as was usual practice in larger slaughterhouses. This practice increased the likelihood of contaminating the meat with infective material. At the time there was no legislation to define best practice. Additionally, large slaughterhouses and meat wholesalers did not use meat from the heads of beasts, nor did they split the skulls to extract the brains.

Further investigations The initial work of the inquiry team found that there was an association between the vCJD cases and the consumption of beef purchased from butchers where meat could have been contaminated with bovine brain. The team interviewed relatives of the victims using a structured questionnaire covering dietary history and the source of the meat likely to have been consumed by the victim during the period from 1980 to 1991 when there was the highest risk of BSE-contaminated meat passing into the food chain. As a control comparison, a relative of each of 30 age-matched individuals, six for each identified case, was interviewed using the same questionnaire.

From the questionnaire, all the possible sources of meat were investigated to try and identify the butchery and slaughter methods used. The result showed that the victims were 15 times more likely to have purchased and consumed beef from a butcher who removed the brain from a beast compared with the control groups who purchased meat from outlets where cross-contamination with brain material was not a risk.

Conclusions Although individuals may not be able to remember where they bought their food or what they fed to their families 20 years ago, the pattern of food purchase, and especially where the meat consumed was sourced, formed a pattern. This pattern indicated for the first time a direct correlation between the meat consumed and the associated butchery and slaughter practice with disease cases. This produced a plausible explanation and correlation of cases and risk. In addition, the careful and exhaustive investigation has identified the likely moment of infection and for the first time has allowed the incubation period in humans of vCJD to be estimated. It is now believed to be within the range of 10–16 years.

Doncaster cluster

Currently there is also an investigation being carried out relating to two deaths, and a possible third, in Armthorpe, near Doncaster. Two of the victims came from the same street, and the third visited the area frequently. Members of the CJD surveillance team have visited the town and inquiries into possible common factors linking the cases are being undertaken. The likely parameters for this and any other investigation have probably been set by the Queniborough cluster.

Prevention of vCJD and BSE

The BSE inquiry[2] stated that government policy was that 'All pathways by which vCJD may be transmitted between humans must be identified and all reasonably practicable measures taken to block them'.

The prevention of the passage of vCJD from sufferers to other humans is addressed in several ways: the World Health Organization (WHO) became involved soon after it became apparent that there might be a link between BSE and the emergence of vCJD. A series of consultations were undertaken with a variety of governmental bodies and eminent scientists. As a result, the WHO made a series of recommendations relating to foodstuffs and product derived from cattle. Milk was considered to be safe; however, tallow and gelatin were only considered to be safe if, during manufacturing, the process involved can inactivate or destroy any prion present. They also recommended that it is important that the pharmaceutical industry obtain bovine materials for use in parenteral, oral or other products from countries which have a surveillance system for BSE in place and which report either no or only sporadic cases of BSE. They also recommended and encouraged the development of diagnostic methods and surveillance to ascertain the spread of CJD.

In the UK regulations have been introduced covering the use of bovine materials in medicines and vaccines. The law came into effect on 1 March 2001 for human medicines, and from 1 June 2001 for veterinary medicines. All manufacturers of licensed medicinal products are affected and the Medicines Control Agency (MCA) and Veterinary Medicines Directorate (VMD) will ensure compliance.[11]

All gelatin, collagen, tallow derivatives, amino acids and peptides made from bovine material and used in the pharmaceutical industry is derived from material obtained from animals slaughtered outside the UK.

Classic CJD has occurred by the transplantation of brain tissue or the use of brain-derived extracts. As a result, surgeons, especially neurosurgeons who treat CJD patients, are advised to destroy all surgical instruments after use. Disposable single-use instruments for tonsillectomies are to be introduced in 2001; the delays in their introduction have led to a backlog of cases awaiting surgery.

Blood and blood products have been identified as carrying a particular risk of transmitting vCJD. Therefore measures have been taken to treat blood used in the UK by leukodepletion to reduce any transmission risk. Fresh frozen human plasma has been imported to produce certain blood products from countries where BSE/vCJD is unknown.[12]

The UK blood transfusion services is informed every 6 months of all definite and probable cases of sporadic and familial CJD who were reported as blood donors and blood product recipients. Whenever a suspected case of vCJD is confirmed as a 'probable' case, comprehensive information is passed to the transfusion service so that any donated blood can be withdrawn, and any blood donors whose blood has been given to the patient traced. Canada and the USA have banned blood donations from people who have spent long periods in the UK, and other countries are considering introducing similar measures.

Prevention strategies

Prevention of a recurrence of the BSE/vCJD outbreak is of paramount importance to the government of the UK, and its subordinate departments. As a result there are several measures which remain in place to reduce the risks of BSE-infected meat entering the human food chain.[13]

Primary prevention focuses on preventing a resurgence of BSE in the UK cattle herd, and the presence of the disease in cattle at slaughter. Additional precautions are aimed at implementing and ensuring good butchery practice.

Any cattle suspected of having BSE are compulsorily slaughtered and their bodies destroyed. Milk produced by cows which are suspected of having BSE may not be used for any purpose other than feeding the cow's own calf. In addition to this very obvious measure there are several other measures in place to protect animal and, by implication, human health.

Beef for human consumption   All cattle reared for beef destined for human consumption have to be slaughtered at an age of less than 30 months. The requirement for removing the bones from meat before retail sale has now been lifted.

The Over Thirty Months Slaughter scheme   The Over Thirty Months Slaughter (OTMS) scheme bans the sale of meat derived from cattle aged over 30 months at the point of slaughter for human consumption and was introduced by SEAC in 1996. At the time of writing this measure is under review by the Food Standards Agency (FSA).

Under the scheme cattle over 30 months of age are purchased, slaughtered and their carcasses incinerated or rendered, and destroyed. This scheme deals with dairy cattle which have reached the end of their productive lactations, old bulls, herd casualties and any other beasts. The animals must have been in the UK for at least 6 months to be eligible. Payment is made on a per kilogram basis as compensation. At June 2000, 4.25 million cattle had been slaughtered under the scheme. Only 403 000 have been incinerated. The other carcasses have been rendered and MBM and tallow are being safely and securely stored awaiting disposal after a safe method is found. New incinerators at Widnes, Wymington and Fawley will join other sites that are burning MBM by April 2001. The Ministry of Agriculture, Fisheries, and Food (MAFF: now the Department for Environment, Food, and Rural Affairs (DEFRA)) expects the backlog of material to be cleared by early 2004.

Due to restrictions on cattle movements imposed during the recent outbreak of foot-and-mouth disease in the UK it is likely that more cattle will enter the OTMS scheme.

Cattle identification and tracing   All cattle born or imported into the UK after September 1998 are registered on a national cattle tracing system managed and operated by DEFRA. All movements of any particular beast are documented from birth until death. Each individual beast has a full passport on which the data are entered. All cattle are also numerically ear-tagged to comply with European Commission regulations, making tracing easier. In the first 6 months of the year 2000, DEFRA, through the British Cattle Movement Service, issued 1 696 010 cattle passports and recorded 3 422 523 cattle movements.

Feed controls   Mammalian-derived meat and bone meal (MMBM) is outlawed from inclusion in ruminant feeds, and all feed mills and farms have had to be cleaned to remove any previous contamination from feed in which MMBM might have been present. A continuing inspection programme is coordinated by DEFRA. Feed is regularly inspected and sampled to ensure compliance.

Bull semen   As mentioned, BSE in cattle is linked to vCJD in humans, and following the identification of maternal spread it soon became apparent that the use of semen from infected bulls could carry a risk that BSE might be introduced into a country or herd of cattle previously certified as disease-free. Following measures instituted by DEFRA to ensure only disease-free semen was available, the export ban of this material was lifted to the European Union in 1996, and to other countries as bilateral agreements were reached based on guarantees of disease-free status. These are now in place with the USA, Canada, South Africa, Australia and New Zealand. The continuance of all these agreements hinges on no cases arising in cattle sired by exported semen, and is an important measure in preventing re-emergence of BSE and thus the risk of infected material reaching the food chain, although current butchery practice would also reduce any risk.

Exported and imported meat   Regulations are now in place which prohibit the export or import of beef, or beef products, which are not certified free of BSE. The penalties and fines applicable to persons or organisations which break the rules are heavy, including fines of up to £5000 and up to 2 years' imprisonment. Any products detected as breaching the regulations are destroyed. Secondary prosecutions in the European Union and other states are also possible. Meat for export must be accompanied by a valid Export Health Certificate, issued in accordance with the provisions of the Products of Animal Origin (Import and Export) Regulations 1992. Heavy fines are imposed for breaches of the regulations in conjunction with destruction of the produce. All exports of beef are deboned before dispatch under the provisions of the Date Based Export Scheme (DBES).

Offspring cull   To arrest the arrival in the adult cattle herd of calves born from cattle diagnosed with BSE, all suspect offspring have to be slaughtered. This eradication and slaughter programme was a prerequisite for the resumption of beef exports from the UK.

Specified risk material   Specified risk material (SRM) is controlled both by law in the UK and under a decision of the European Commission in Europe. The UK has a higher standard of exclusion than the European Commission on this matter and excludes more material from inclusion. Pithing is also to be outlawed both within the European Community and also by import control in all countries wishing to export to the European Community. The measures aim to prevent material entering not only the human food chain but also animal feed, fertiliser or other cattle-derived materials. SRM may not be fed to any animal, nor may MMBM be incorporated in agricultural fertiliser. Controls on SRM prohibit the use of certain specified animal products which are known to harbour, or might theoretically harbour, BSE infectivity.

Scrapie   Scrapie in sheep is still seen as the original source of BSE, and thus vCJD in humans. DEFRA has agreed the proposal by SEAC for a National Scrapie Plan, which aims to develop a programme to control and eradicate the disease. The initial measures proposed include ram genotyping to prevent the siring of susceptible or infected breed stock. Legislation measures which came into effect on 1 July 1998 made it compulsory to slaughter all sheep and goats displaying clinical signs of scrapie. A compensation scheme is in place, and it is the responsibility of DEFRA to dispose of the carcasses and keep statistics.

The future for vCJD

It is uncertain what the future will hold. Estimates vary from the condition reaching epidemic proportions, with mass fatalities, to suggestions that, although there will continue to be a trickle of confirmed cases annually, widespread fatality is unlikely. As with many other issues, our knowledge will develop with the passage of time, as will any cases currently in incubation. As my grandmother always said: 'them that lives the longest, will see the most'.

Useful addresses

The National CJD Surveillance Unit
Western General Hospital
Crewe Road
Edinburgh EH4 2XU
Tel: +44 (0)131 332 2117
Fax: +44 (0)131 343 1404

Prion Disease Group
Department of Neurogenics
Imperial College School of Medicine
St Mary's Campus
Norfolk Place
London W2 1PG

Tel: +44 (0)20 7594 3760
Fax: +44 (0)20 7706 7094

CJD Support Network
Birchwood Heath Top
Ashley Heath Market
Drayton
Salop TF9 4QR
Tel: +44 (0)1630 673993
Helpline: +44 (0)1630 673973

References

1. Public Health Laboratory Service. *Statutory Notifications of Infectious Diseases; Notifications of Food Poisoning.* London: PHLS, 2001.
2. Anonymous. *Report of the BSE Inquiry.* London: Stationery Office, 2000.
3. Anonymous. *BSE in Great Britain: A Progress Report.* London: Ministry of Agriculture, Fisheries, and Food, 2000.
4. Budka H, Aguzzi A, Brown P, *et al.* Tissue handling in suspected Creutzfeldt–Jakob disease (CJD) and other human spongiform encephalopathies (prion diseases). *Brain Pathol* 1995; 5: 319–322.
5. Will R G, Ironside J W, Zeidler M, *et al.* A new variant of Creutzfeldt–Jakob disease in the UK. *Lancet* 1996; 347: 921–925.
6. Will R G, Stewart G, Zeidler M, *et al.* Psychiatric features of new variant Creutzfeldt–Jakob disease. *Psychol Bull* 1999; 23: 264–267.
7. MacLeod M A, Knight R, Stewart G, *et al.* Sensory features of variant Creutzfeldt–Jakob disease. *J Neurol Neurosurg Psychiatry* 2000; 69: 413–414.
8. Macleod M A, Knight R, Stewart G, *et al.* Clinical features of nvCJD. *Eur J Neurol* 1999; 6: 26–27.
9. Will R G, Zeidler M, Stewart G E, *et al.* Diagnosis of new variant Creutzfeldt–Jakob disease. *Ann Neurol* 2000; 47: 575–582.
10. Campbell H, Douglas M J, Will R J. Patients with new variant Creutzfeldt–Jakob disease and their families: care and information needs. Creutzfeldt–Jakob Disease Study Unit: http://www.cjd.ed.ac.uk February 1999.
11. Minor P D, Will R G, Salisbury D. Vaccines and variant CJD. *Vaccine* 2000; 19: 409–410.
12. Turner M. Universal leucodepletion to reduce potential risk of transmission of new-variant Creutzfeldt–Jakob disease. *Br J Haematol* 2000; 110: 745–747.
13. Anonymous. BSE and vCJD: causes, controls and concerns. *Vet Rec* 2000; 147: 405–406.

6

Pandora's box

Pandora was the first woman to be created. She was fashioned from clay
by Hephaestus at the request of Zeus. The gods gave her every advantage
they were able to grant. Zeus then gave her a box to present to the man
who married her. He planned to destroy man, who had been created
by Prometheus, by giving the man Pandora as a wife. Knowing that
Prometheus would be too wise to accept the gift, Zeus persuaded his
less cautious brother Epimetheus to marry her. Later Pandora, against
the instructions of the gods, opened the box and let loose upon
the world all evils and diseases. In the bottom of the box only Hope
remained.

Ancient Greek myth

Most of the zoonoses already discussed in this volume lead to death
only in an infected human following a prolonged untreated infection.
The zoonoses discussed in this chapter are less benign, and entirely more
sinister. Their very names – anthrax, Ebola, plague and rabies – carry an
echo of unspeakable evil. This may only be a fantasy or a folk memory,
yet the facts speak for themselves. Once infected, the chance of mortality with any of these agents is much higher than with other zoonoses,
especially if treatment is delayed once symptoms appear.

Having been demonised by our media in books, films and newspapers (the image of Dustin Hoffmann fighting against an epidemic of
massive mortality in *Outbreak* is an enduring one for all who have seen
it), where does the truth lie? This chapter sets out to answer some of the
following questions: how dangerous are these infections? What are the
mortality statistics? What are the available treatments, if any?

Although not endemic in the UK, all of these diseases could appear
here carried by fomites, animals or humans, depending on their mechanism of spread. If robust measures were not put in place rapidly on the
appearance of an initial case, a pestilence of biblical proportions could
ensue. It is not for nothing that one of the horsemen of the apocalypse
is named as pestilence or plague.

As has been mentioned in Chapter 1, our temperate climate,
geographical isolation and quarantine system give the UK a degree of

protection against the more dramatic manifestations of serious zoonoses. The system of quarantine certainly has afforded us comprehensive protection against rabies for many years, and the advent of a well-regulated system of pet passports is unlikely to compromise that system. In contrast, we cannot quarantine human beings except in rare and exceptional circumstances. Not all immigrants to our country – be they animal or human – stop at the immigration office on the way in, nor can we tell if they are infected if they do. Migrating birds are believed to have been responsible for the outbreak of West Nile virus in New York which killed eight people between September 2000 and September 2001. They do not stop at borders for a health check.

Historically, the bubonic plague was introduced into the country by rats from ships, and the epidemiology of the Black Death began with the first cases being seen at Melcombe in Dorset. The likelihood of a recurrence of plague from such a source is reduced by inspections and mandatory fumigation of vessels as well as the system of public health measures aimed at controlling the rodent populations. Nevertheless there still remains a risk, and the price of safety is constant vigilance. Part of any system of vigilance has to be the education of healthcare professionals in the signs and symptoms associated with these diseases and this chapter aims to forward that objective.

It is not only animals and humans that travel today; goods are transported from far and near to fuel the appetite of our domestic market. Fomites transfer or objects contaminated with spores are particularly important in the transmission of anthrax. Recently the importation by both tourists and commercial companies of items made from goatskins in Haiti and the Dominican Republic has been banned as these items have been shown to be contaminated with anthrax spores.

There is another dimension to several of the diseases examined in this section. Biological warfare has been the subject of a wide debate in modern society. It has a long and less than glorious history linking the catapulting of dead animals and humans into besieged strongholds by our ancestors to the possibility of Scud missiles loaded with anthrax being fired from Iraq into Israel. Biological warfare is banned by international treaty, and enforced by United Nation inspection. However, as recent events in the USA have shown, this is not sufficient to prevent individuals or states pursuing this route in the hope of causing megadeath to their adversaries. Some of the organisms discussed in this chapter have the potential to be biological agents for weapons of mass destruction. This also helps link these zoonoses in readers' minds with the everyday world of media reportage and will perhaps dispel some of the wilder journalistic assertions.[1]

Anthrax
(Malignant pustule, woolsorter's disease, charbon, malignant oedema, splenic fever)

Anthrax is an acute bacterial disease of animals and humans which can cause rapid fatality (hence the old English name of 'struck' for the disease in cattle). It is caused by *Bacillus anthracis*, a Gram-positive, encapsulated, spore-forming bacterium which spores rapidly on contact with oxygen. When cultured it produces dense colonies on agar with long chains of bacteria forming so-called 'medusa-head colonies' from their shape and appearance.

This disease occurs worldwide and is an occupational hazard for those involved in processing the wool, hide, hair or bones of animals, such as farmers, slaughterers, skinners, hideworkers, tanners and woolworkers. Most mammals are susceptible to the disease. It is most commonly seen in cattle; goats, sheep, horses and pigs can also contract the disease.

Anthrax is a notifiable disease in the UK. Notification also applies to animals suspected of having died of the disease. Carcasses must be disposed of by burning or by liming followed by deep burial. Definitive diagnosis is not always possible as opening or moving suspect carcasses is also prohibited.

Luckily, the disease is rare in the UK. The most recent case occurred in August 2000 in Bradford after a man involved in the wool trade was diagnosed as having the cutaneous form. After treatment he survived.[2]

Many of the non-fatal cases in the USA associated with the handling of contaminated mail have also been of the cutaneous form.

An outbreak in 1979 at Sverdlosk, Russia, seems to have been related to an accidental release from a biological weapons research facility. Sixty-six people died, although the authorities claim that the cases resulted from the ingestion of poorly cooked infected meat.[3]

A large outbreak in Zimbabwe from October 1979 to March 1980 caused more than 6000 (mostly cutaneous) cases. In Paraguay 25 cutaneous cases were seen in 1987 following the slaughter of an infected cow. Currently the Department of Health (DoH) considers South and Central America, southern and eastern Europe, Asia, Africa, the Caribbean and the Middle East as areas where the disease may occur in significant amounts.

Disease in animals

Anthrax in animals often follows the grazing of pasture infected with viable spores. The spores are resistant to a wide range of climatic conditions and can remain in contaminated ground for many years. In one reported incident from Hawaii, a cow died after grazing a pasture where the carcass of a cow suspected of having died of the disease 20 years previously was buried. Animals may also demonstrate in-species spread from infected meat or by close contact with an infected beast.

Symptoms in animals are usually acute, with high fever of sudden onset, localised swellings and profuse bleeding from orifices. Death usually occurs 24–72 hours after onset. Animals may be found dead or moribund.

Transmission

The spores present in the animal's blood or secretions, infected pastures, hides and bone or meat. Transmission to humans follows contact with these spores.

Disease in humans

The disease presents in distinct forms in humans depending on the route of infection. These are:

1. Cutaneous, following physical contact with spores and their subsequent inoculation into wounds or abrasions.
2. Pulmonary, following inhalation of spores from infected hides.
3. Intestinal, following ingestion of spores or organism in undercooked meat from infected carcasses.

Infected individuals display the disease after a variable incubation period depending on route of infection. The cutaneous form develops after 2–10 days, the pulmonary after 1–5 days and the intestinal after 2–5 days.

The cutaneous form, once known as malignant pustule, is responsible for 98% of cases worldwide. After the incubation period, a papular spot develops on the skin. This papule becomes vesicular and turns black in the centre. This forms an eschar (a plug of dead tissue, skin and blood) which causes necrosis of the underlying tissue and then sloughs off. There is very little pain or tenderness associated with the condition, although local lymph nodes usually swell. Extensive oedema affecting the whole limb or upper body is often seen and is important in differentiating the disease from tick-borne disease where an eschar may also be present. Some patients will display fever, lethargy, sickness and severe headache. The skin lesion will often heal without treatment, but there is a 5–20% risk of untreated cases progressing to septicaemia or meningitis with fatal consequences after the eschar sloughs. Cutaneous spread to other people is possible.

Pulmonary anthrax, known as woolsorter's disease, follows inhalation of spores from infected hides or wool. It presents as a flu-like illness after the incubation period, followed by cough and severe shortness of breath. This develops into respiratory failure and can be fatal within 24 hours, usually following septicaemic spread.

All of the fatal cases seen in the US terrorist attacks during 2001 have been from the pulmonary form. Prior to the extensive number of cases seen, this form of the disease was believed to be fatal in all cases regardless of the rapidity with which treatment was commenced. This has proved erroneous, with death only occurring in 40% of cases.[4] There are still no known cases stemming from pulmonary spread from existing patients to other individuals, although precautions have been taken to prevent such an eventuality.

Intestinal anthrax follows ingestion of infected meat. The rarity of the condition is related to the low incidence of the disease in meat in developed countries, and the unlikely nature of ingesting enough viable spores or organisms to cause disease.

Severe copious diarrhoea occurs after the incubation period. Half of untreated cases will die.

Diagnosis

Identifying the causative organism in blood smears makes the diagnosis. Growing samples on standard culture media leads to the development of characteristic colonies, with the bacterium showing centrally placed spores. Immunofluorescent and enzyme-linked immunosorbent assay (ELISA) techniques can also be used.

Treatment

Anthrax is susceptible to most common antibiotics. There are reports of rare strains being found which are resistant to either penicillin or doxycycline.[5]

Drug regimes culled from the literature include: Benzlpenicillin (penicillin G) 2 million units (IU) intravenously every 4 hours, tetracycline 500 mg by mouth 6-hourly, ciprofloxacin 400 mg intravenously every 12 hours or doxycycline 100 mg intravenously every 12 hours. There is little clinical experience with these regimes, although they have been used experimentally in laboratories. Therefore they must be treated with some caution, except for the penicillin dose regime.[6, 7]

Prevention

A vaccine derived from a cell-free filtrate of killed bacteria is available and licensed for human use in the UK. Supplies are kept by the Public Health Laboratory Service (PHLS), and are usually issued for use in workers considered to be at a high occupational risk. The vaccination regime consists of three doses given over a period of 6 weeks with a booster dose given after 6 months. An annual booster is necessary to maintain immunity. A vaccine is also available for animals, but it is only for emergency use and is obtained through the Ministry of Agriculture, Fisheries, and Food (MAFF: now the Department for Environment, Food, and Rural Affairs (DEFRA)).

Prophylactic use of antibiotics may also be appropriate. The *British National Formulary* (*BNF*)[8] has no recommendations; in contrast, in the American literature drugs of choice are tetracyclines, including doxycycline and ciprofloxacin. The recommended regimes are doxycycline 100 mg every 12 hours by mouth, ciprofloxacin 500 mg by mouth 12-hourly. Due to the persistence of spores in tissues following contact with dense inocula, it may be necessary to continue prophylaxis for 4–6 weeks after exposure. Vaccination may be necessary during antibiotic prophylaxis to give protection after discontinuing the drug therapy.

Physical prevention methods are based on preventing or limiting contact with infected animals or their hides, hair or meat. All surface wounds should be disinfected and covered. Physical disinfection of hides and hair is considered to be good practice in the tanning and wool industry. The use of formaldehyde as a disinfectant is carried out by specialist companies for imports of hide, bones and bone meal (much reduced in volume since the advent of bovine spongiform encephalopathy (BSE)) and wool. Heat treatment is also used. Animals suspected of having died of the disease are to be handled in accordance with biohazard procedures. Suitable protective clothing and filtered ventilation helmets should be worn.

Spores may be killed by heat with autoclaving or boiling infected materials or instruments where appropriate. In areas where anthrax is endemic, meat should be thoroughly cooked or avoided.

Formaldehyde and glutaraldehyde are effective disinfectants for dealing with local contamination and spillages, though it is recommended that clothing and other articles of victims should be incinerated carefully.

Potential as a biological warfare agent

Anthrax can be cultured successfully and its spores harvested. The spores can then be turned into a dry powder. During the First World War, the Germans produced sugar lumps inoculated with anthrax for feeding to allied draught horses. There were also incidents of bags of powder containing anthrax spores being dropped from German aircraft. In 1942–1943, the British conducted trials on Gruinard Island off the north-west coast of Scotland to investigate the feasibility of biological warfare using anthrax. (The island was finally declared safe in 1990.) In an associated programme, the UK developed cattle cakes inoculated with anthrax for retaliatory strikes against Germany. These were to have been dropped from bomber aircraft in the event of a German strike. In Germany warheads containing anthrax were developed for attachment to V1 and V2 weapons. The escalation of hostilities that such weapons would have caused led to neither side employing them offensively.[7]

In Japan during the 1990s, the Aum Shinrikyo cult released anthrax spores in Tokyo. Luckily there were no fatalities. Following the Iran–Iraq war and the Gulf War, Iraq was shown to have produced shells and missile warheads packed with spores.

Many authorities view anthrax as the greatest threat for use in biological warfare or terrorism. With the cases caused by contaminated mail in the USA in the aftermath of the events of September the 11th, it has become apparent that as a terrorist weapon it has a tremendous potential to cause widespread concern with some fatalities, even when the potency has not been enhanced by finely grinding the powder containing the spores.

Ebola
(African haemorrhagic fever; Ebola haemorrhagic fever)

Ebola is probably one of the most emotive and dramatic zoonotic infections. It is caused by a virus similar in form to Marburg virus but distinguished by differences in antigen testing profile. The virus is named after a river in the Democratic Republic of the Congo (formerly Zaire). Classified as an RNA filovirus, it shows strange branching and filamentous forms displayed by no other viral group. There are four subtypes of the virus. The three demonstrated to be pathogenic in humans are Ebola–Ivory Coast, Ebola–Sudan, and Ebola–Zaire. The fourth, Ebola–Reston, has been shown to be pathogenic in apes but not for infected humans. This last type was identified in monkeys imported from the Philippines into Italy and North America for laboratory use. Several research workers became infected with the virus, although none became ill.[9]

Ebola haemorrhagic fever was first recognised in 1976, when large outbreaks occurred in southern Sudan and neighbouring northern Zaire. Since then it has appeared sporadically in these and other areas of Africa. There has been only one case recorded outside Africa with a single non-fatal case in a laboratory in the UK following a needlestick injury. The pathogenic forms of the virus are not known to be native to other continents.

Transmission

The natural reservoir of Ebola virus is unknown at present. It has been postulated that the natural reservoir could be bats. Recently scientists from the Institut Pasteur, Paris, have detected it in small rodents in the Central African Republic.[10] There is still work to be done to discover how the rodents transmit the virus to apes and monkeys which have previously been identified as the link to human infection. The handling of ill or dead infected chimpanzees was shown to be the source of human infection in the outbreaks in the Ivory Coast and Gabon.

The main concern for countries outside Africa stems from the latent period of the infection. In theory it would be possible for an infected individual to carry the disease into a city or country where unrecognised the disease could rapidly spread. Mortality rates have been as high as 90% in some outbreaks so the fear is not unfounded.

Disease in humans

The virus has an incubation period of between 2 and 21 days after exposure and infection in humans before clinical signs are seen. Weakness and lethargy follow a sudden onset of fever with a temperature as high as 39°C. Muscle and joint pain are seen in most cases, with sore throat, headache and occasionally hiccups. More severe symptoms follow with anorexia, nausea, vomiting and diarrhoea. The development of a severe skin rash and mental confusion is concurrent with the progression of the illness. Kidney and liver damage occurs and catastrophic internal and external haemorrhage leads to death towards the beginning of the second week. The virus is present in high concentrations in the blood, tissue fluids and most organs of the body. Patients lucky enough to survive require extended periods of care.

Human-to-human transmission occurs following direct contact with the blood, secretions or semen of infected patients. Following the first confirmed or index case transmission occurs to those in closest contact with the victim. These can be friends, family or healthcare workers. Nosocomial spread or spread from a clinic or hospital to staff or other patients has occurred several times in major outbreaks, leading to high mortality rates. In Africa limitations on availability of disposable equipment and protective clothing have also led to transmission. The disease can also be sexually transmitted through semen up to 7 weeks after clinical recovery. All Ebola virus subtypes have displayed the ability to be spread through aerosols under research conditions, although aerosol spread has not been demonstrated during outbreaks.

Outbreak statistics

Between June and November 1976 the Ebola virus infected 284 people in Sudan, with 117 deaths. During the outbreaks 76 of the 230 staff at Maridi Hospital contracted Ebola fever, with 41 subsequently dying. In Zaire there were 318 cases and 280 deaths in September and October 1976.

There was an isolated case in Zaire in 1977 and a second outbreak in Sudan in 1979. One human case of Ebola haemorrhagic fever and several cases in chimpanzees were confirmed in the Ivory Coast in 1994 when a scientist contracted the disease after conducting an autopsy on a wild chimpanzee found dead with signs of haemorrhagic disease. Fortune favours the foolish and the brave and he spontaneously recovered.

In Gabon, Ebola haemorrhagic fever was first documented in 1994 and two outbreaks occurred in February 1996 and July 1996, with 37 cases and 21 deaths in Makokou, related to cooking a chimpanzee and 61 cases and 45 deaths in Booue.

A large epidemic occurred in Kikwit, Zaire, in 1995 with 315 cases, 244 of whom died. This outbreak was thought to have occurred after the index case handled a monkey and smoked its flesh.

Ebola virus infections were not reported again until the autumn of 2000 when an outbreak occurred in the Gulu district of northern Uganda. This is the first outbreak ever documented in Uganda. As of 19 December 2000, the Ugandan Ministry of Health reported cumulative figures for all affected districts of 421 cases, including 162 deaths. Spread had been dramatic both in the community and hospitals, with healthcare workers amongst the dead.[11]

The outbreak was finally declared over by the World Health Organization (WHO) at the end of February 2001.[12] The final official death toll was 224. Including this outbreak, there have been approximately 1500 cases with over 1000 fatalities since the identification of the virus.

Treatment

There is no therapeutic treatment for the disease. Supportive measures, such as rehydration by intravenous fluids, blood transfusion, use of nutritional supplements (again by intravenous route) and management of kidney failure, can improve the outcome of the disease. Rapid treatment of secondary infections is also very important, especially in the convalescent patient. During the Kikwit outbreak in 1995, eight patients were given blood donated by survivors. Seven of the eight patients recovered, probably as a result of the conferred immunity, although this treatment has not been properly clinically evaluated.

Prevention

Any imported apes which have not been bred in captivity must be strictly quarantined. For best practice this should be extended to all primates, as the Ebola–Reston variety was found in apes previously held in a facility in Manila where fresh-caught and captive-bred apes were mixed.

Strict hygiene measures should be employed. Appropriate protective clothing should be worn at all times.

Suspected Ebola haemorrhagic fever is a notifiable disease in the UK, both domestically and to the World Health Organization (WHO). For healthcare workers strict barrier nursing and the use and careful disposal of gloves, syringes, needles and dressings are essential. All clinical specimens have to be handled according to guidelines for extremely hazardous substances. Immediate disposal of bodies in secure body bags with prompt burial or cremation is necessary during an outbreak.

Case contacts or individuals exposed in laboratories must be placed under health surveillance for 3 weeks after their last possible exposure to infection. If there is the onset of febrile symptoms they must be placed in strict isolation until diagnostic test results are obtained.

In Africa, as the infection route is still unclear, prevention of Ebola poses a major problem. Educating healthcare workers and others to identify a suspected case early and to be able to isolate the patient with appropriate barrier nursing techniques is seen as the main thrust of current limitation strategies. The main obstacle to the success of such a strategy is the availability of sterile materials, protective clothing and appropriate facilities. Usually once a case has been confirmed by diagnostic tests an outbreak is already underway.

Plague
(The Black Death, bubonic and pneumonic plague)

Any book about zoonoses would not be complete without a section on plague, and any section on plague must detail the historic importance of the ravages associated with the disease. Even today, it is not unusual to see children in the playground singing and acting out 'Ring-a-ring o'roses, a pocket full of posies, a-tishoo, a-tishoo, we all fall down'. This anonymous nursery rhyme, originating in the middle of the 17th century, is a graphic and simple representation of the effects of an outbreak of pneumonic plague. The importance of rat control is emphasised in the same way, with the telling of the tale of the Pied Piper of Hamelin.

Historians differ in their view of the worst results of epidemic plague, and the numbers of casualties quoted for pandemics are probably in legal terms 'unsafe'. The widest geographic epidemics are usually known as pandemics and the consensus of opinion is that in recorded history there have been three outbreaks which could be thus classified.

The first to spread across Europe started in the 6th century, and was known as the Plague of Justinian. There were widespread fatalities. This outbreak was seen as a visitation by God on a sinful people; however, the religiosity it engendered was no protection against flea bites and disease.

The outbreak now termed the Second Pandemic or the Black Death started from a natural focus somewhere in Mesopotamia in western Turkey during the 11th century. Plague-infected rats and their associated fleas, carried aboard trading ships, spread the Black Death from Tana in the Crimea, Ukraine, to Messina in Sicily in 1347. In the ensuing European plague, which endured up to the end of the 17th century, it is variously estimated that a quarter to a half of the population died as a result of this disease alone. At the height of the epidemic in the 14th century, the effect upon all aspects of social and international development was profound: large swathes of land in Europe became uninhabited. The epidemic in the UK in the 1660s, which caused the Plague of London and other local outbreaks, stemmed from this pandemic. Although important in British history, it was insignificant in world terms, with only 70 000 fatalities.

The third and last pandemic occurred during the late 19th century. It owed its rapid spread to commercial shipping, with infected rats becoming stowaways on fast steam packets leaving Hong Kong and Canton in 1894 for many other ports the world over. Within a decade it had spread to over 70 ports on five continents. Coming as it did at a time when scientific endeavour and disciplines were developing, the bacterium, its association with rats and the rat flea as a vector were soon identified, allowing prevention strategies to be put in place.

The disease

The pathogen responsible for plague is *Yersinia pestis*, a Gram-negative coccobacillus. A facultative anaerobe, the bacterium is capable of forming an encapsulated spore swiftly when exposed to the air. The risk of infection from the spores, which are able to survive under suitable conditions for prolonged periods of time, has been considered a significant risk in archaeological excavations of burial sites.

During the Second World War, part of the Blitz upon London was aimed at disturbing the plague pits used for burials during the Plague of London three centuries previously, in the hope of releasing viable spores into the environment. Had this succeeded, the death toll from this disease, let loose in a city with increasing rodent numbers, poor sanitation and a displaced human population, would doubtless have been high.

This was not the first use of the disease as a weapon of war. Corpses of humans and animals which had died of this and other diseases have in the past been hurled into besieged cities using catapults. This stratagem was used in the hope and certainty of infecting the garrison from the earliest recorded incidents of siege warfare until modern times. In 1346 a Tartar army besieging the city of Kaffa, in what is now Turkey, suffered from plague. They threw their dead into the city over the walls, and the resulting epidemic forced the defenders to surrender.

Plague has been identified as a pathogen at the centre of several countries' programmes of biological warfare development. Russia is known to have a genetically manipulated strain, designed for use. Both North Korea and Israel are known to have studied the use of this pathogen extensively in an offensive military role. If employed, the pathogen would be delivered using an air-borne route, so giving pneumonic plague to victims.

Wild foci

Wild plague foci, where suitable rodent populations and habitat conditions exist, are found in the western USA, some countries in South America, extensive areas of north-central, eastern and southern Africa, Madagascar, Iran, and also along the frontier between Yemen and Saudi Arabia, Central and South-east Asia, and portions of the Former Soviet Union[13] (Figure 6.1).

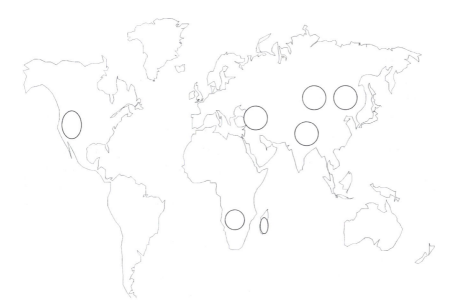

Figure 6.1   Sylvatic (wild) plague foci across the world. Data from Dennis *et al.*[14]

These foci are associated with dry areas, usually where desert or prairie-type landscapes form. Foci are normally away from urban areas because of their inaccessibility, or their inhospitable nature. It is therefore unusual to find human cases emanating from wild foci sources; however, in the USA where there has been rapid expansion of urban areas and isolated condominium building, an increasing number of human cases come from this source.

Rodents in a natural plague focus become immune to the disease. However, if they spread from the focus into another distinct rodent population, especially one linked to an urbanised site, infection of a susceptible population of rodents may produce massive fatalities. This can lead to the phenomenon known as rat-fall, where a large number of rodent corpses are seen in open areas. Associated with this event are usually reports of fleas biting humans: the rat fleas leave the corpses in search of new hosts, and this results in disease transfer.

The world picture

The WHO made the latest worldwide study of plague in 1997. In that year there were 5419 cases of the disease reported, with 274 deaths. More than 70% of cases were in Africa and the country with the highest number was Madagascar, with more than half of the reported total occurring there. Interestingly, there has been a small but steady rise of numbers of cases annually since the mid 1980s. This may be due to a true increase in cases, or just better detection and reporting. Plague is one of only three infectious diseases subject to the International Health Regulations. All confirmed cases should be reported to the WHO.[14]

In Africa, plague was reported from six countries – Madagascar, Malawi, Mozambique, Tanzania, Zambia and Zimbabwe. The total number of cases in 1997 was 5101, with 261 fatalities. Of these, 2863 were reported from Madagascar, with 176 deaths.

The whole of the American continent – Central, North and South America – only reported 44 cases in 1997. Bolivia reported a single case, Peru had 39 cases and the USA reported four cases, with one being fatal. The cases were reported from Arizona, Colorado and California.

Five Asian nations reported 274 cases, with 12 fatalities. These were in China, Indonesia, Kazakhstan, Mongolia and Vietnam. China had 43 cases, Indonesia six, Kazakhstan one, Mongolia four, Vietnam 220. Of the deaths, 10 were in Vietnam. It is possible that reporting from these countries might be incomplete.

Epidemiology

In terms of the development of an epidemic, the re-emergence of plague in India in 1994 after a gap of reported cases of nearly 30 years is interesting. In 1993 a severe earthquake hit areas previously identified as having wild plague foci. The resulting devastation allowed the rat population to increase dramatically, with a corresponding increase in the population of their associated fleas. In August 1994 a village in the Beed district reported rat-fall and subsequent flea nuisance. An outbreak of bubonic plague followed, with 596 cases but no fatalities.

A separate outbreak in Gujarat followed flooding associated with a record monsoon rainfall. During the clean-up operation, workers came into contact with infected animal corpses. The initial cases turned into secondary pneumonic plague, and subsequently, during an influx of people into Surat City for a religious festival, an outbreak of pneumonic plague ensued. Of 151 cases, 52 died.

The area of most concern in plague infection is currently Madagascar. A strain of *Y. pestis* showing multiple antibiotic resistance has emerged there.[15] The island has an unusual animal population: rodent species are widespread, leading to an atypical pattern of foci with a higher risk to the human population. The majority of cases are bubonic, due to the virtually universal source of infection being primary contact with rodent fleas.[16]

Disease in animals

The primary wildlife reservoirs of plague are rodent species. The rat, either the domestic black rat (*Rattus rattus*) or the urban brown rat (*R. norvegicus*), is the most important reservoir and rodent vector. Other species may be involved depending on the site and situation of the natural foci involved. Under the normal circumstances in a natural wild focus, the disease cycles within the rodent population and is transferred by fleas which are often specific to the rodent species involved (Figure 6.2).

Other animal species capable of carrying, amplifying or transmitting plague include goats, dogs, cats, squirrels, camels and rabbits. Dogs usually have a brief illness and often recover; cats are not so fortunate. They will often have severe fatal infection with high fever, swollen lymph nodes, pneumonic symptoms and encephalitis. Cats have caused human infection, usually following bites or scratches or inhalation by the human of aerosolised cat secretions. Other non-rodent species are also theoretically able to infect humans via similar routes.

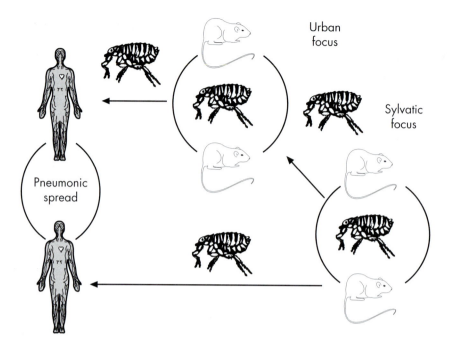

Figure 6.2 Plague cycle from sylvatic (wild) focus to urban rodent focus and humans.

Transmission

The infection of the first, and sometimes only, victim in an outbreak can almost be classed as accidental, following bites from rodent fleas, either in a natural focus or following a rat-fall. The infection may also follow direct contact with rodents, especially if they are butchered or skinned. The route of infection under these circumstances can be by direct transfer of blood, ingestion of infected tissue or inhalation of infected aerosols of blood or mucus. There is some evidence that fomites spread by knives or other instruments used to slaughter or butcher rodents is also possible.

Once an infected host has been bitten, the bacterium is ingested and multiplies in the flea's gut. The bacterium secretes a coagulase, causing an occlusive clot to form in the mid-gut of the flea. This causes blood from a previous bite to be regurgitated during the next bite, due to the obstruction, and the structure of the flea's mouth parts. Inevitably this leads to transfer of the bacteria in the most efficient manner possible. Once infected, fleas can remain infective for a period of weeks or months. The coagulated mass can also ultimately kill the flea. The inoculum necessary to initiate clinical disease, if delivered by the bite of a flea, is believed to be a single viable organism.[17]

The usual route of infection for humans is by rat flea bite. There have also been cases of plague being transmitted from human to human via the bite of a human flea. This is believed to be extremely rare.

Disease in humans

The course that the disease then takes depends upon the route of infection and the symptoms displayed. Cases are classified as bubonic, septicaemic, meningeal, pharyngeal or pneumonic plague.

Bubonic plague

This is the classic pattern of infection following the bites of infected fleas or inoculation of a wound with contaminated material. Following infection, an incubation period of 2–6 days is normally seen. As with many other diseases, the initial signs and symptoms following inoculation can be very generalised and non-specific, but with an acute onset. A fever with headache, chills, fatigue, sickness, joint pain and sore throat are the first clinical signs, indistinguishable from infection with other pathogens.

Following these initial symptoms, and with persistent fever which may increase, there is a progressive swelling of the lymph nodes. This usually commences with the node nearest the site of inoculation. The nodes become tender and are known as buboes, hence the condition's name. Vomiting and muscle pain with delirium usually follow. The swollen nodes fill with pus and the disease spreads, both through the lymphatic system and the blood stream. The skin over the node becomes reddened, shiny and swollen.

On treatment the reddening starts to resolve. However the buboes, especially the first, only subside over a period of time. The initial site can remain swollen for weeks and may require surgical removal for full recovery to take place. In untreated cases, more than half of patients will die.

Septicaemic plague

Primary septicaemic plague does not present with a bubo. There is a high fever, with gastrointestinal disturbance. Symptoms may be confused with urinary tract or chest infections, appendicitis or a viral infection. Pneumonic plague may develop. The disease is progressive, and mediated by an endotoxin secreted by the pathogen. There is an overwhelming immunological response, resulting in a type of anaphylactic shock. Intravascular coagulation may occur with multiple organ failure and respiratory distress, thrombosis and subdermal haemorrhage leading to the blackening and focal necrosis (the symptom from which the soubriquet 'Black Death' comes) of the skin. Meningeal plague can be present, as can ophthalmic involvement and hepatic or splenic abscesses.

Meningeal plague

Usually seen as a complication of bubonic or septicaemic plague, it can also be a primary infection. Fever, headache, stiffness of the neck, with increasing delirium and confusion followed by coma are normally seen. The pathogen can be isolated from cerebrospinal fluid. Most cases follow delayed, inappropriate or bacteriostatic antibiotic therapy. The use of any antibiotic incapable of crossing the blood–brain barrier carries with it the risk of developing this form of disease.

Pharyngeal plague

Pharyngeal plague follows inhalation and deposition in the nose, mouth or throat of large droplets of infected pulmonary exudate or ingestion of infected raw or undercooked meat. Clinical signs mimic bacterial or viral pharyngitis, with severe lymph node swellings. The only way of characterising the infection and the responsible pathogen is by identification from a throat swab and subsequent culture. The course of the disease is variable; however, it normally progresses to a bubonic infection if the patient survives for long.

Pneumonic plague

Patients suffering from bubonic or septicaemic plague may have a dissemination of infection to form a focus in the lungs, known as secondary pneumonic infection. Although their infection remains mainly bubonic, and the clinical course is relatively unaltered, they can develop cough with production of aerosolised infected pulmonary exudate. This can transfer infections to other individuals who then develop a primary pneumonic form of the disease. Once individuals display pneumonic symptoms they are extremely contagious and the spread of the disease within human outbreaks is usually by this rapid route, without the further involvement of rodents or fleas. For the infection to spread, other individuals need to be within 2 m of an actively coughing patient.

Humid overcrowded living areas encourage and promote human-to-human spread.

Pneumonic plague is the form of the disease associated with the highest rate of fatality. The prepatent period is very short: 24–72 hours after exposure. The initial symptoms are similar to other forms of the disease but there is marked physical weakness and respiratory difficulty. A productive cough with copious thin sputum, gradually increasing chest pain, breathing difficulties and the coughing of blood are progressive signs as the condition worsens. Deterioration is very rapid and death occurs within 3 days in almost all untreated patients.

To avert this outcome, antibiotic therapy must be commenced within 18–24 hours of clinical onset. Development of concurrent septicaemic plague and associated complications make supportive therapy and nursing difficult.

Diagnosis

The WHO recommends that immediately a diagnosis of human plague is suspected on clinical and epidemiological grounds, appropriate specimens for diagnosis should be obtained and the patient should be started on specific antimicrobial therapy without waiting for laboratory results. Victims suspected of having the pneumonic form should be placed in isolation wards and barrier-nursed.

Confirmation of the diagnosis follows isolation, culture and identification of *Y. pestis* from specimens. Staining with Wayson or Giemsa stain leaves the pathogen showing a distinctive bipolar appearance. On microscopic examination they have a distinctive 'safety-pin' shape. Serological testing, ELISA and antibody testing can also be used if available. In some cases, diagnosis is only confirmed retrospectively by autopsy.

Treatment

The first response to plague infection is antibiotics. The following notes come from various WHO documents. Any cases seen in the UK would be treated at specialist level, therefore the notes are here for information only and included for the sake of completeness.

The aminoglycosides: streptomycin and gentamicin

Streptomycin is the most effective antibiotic against *Y. pestis* and the drug of choice for treatment of plague, particularly the pneumonic form. Therapeutic effect may be expected with 30 mg/kg per day (up to a total of 2 g/day) in divided doses given intramuscularly, to be continued for a full course of 10 days of therapy or until 3 days after the temperature has returned to normal. Gentamicin can be used at doses of 3 mg/kg per day in adults, 6–7.5 mg/kg per day in children, and 7.5 mg/kg per day in infants.[14]

Chloramphenicol

Chloramphenicol is a suitable alternative to aminoglycosides in the treatment of bubonic or septicaemic plague and is the drug of choice for treatment of patients with meningeal, ophthalmic or pleural complications. A dose of 50 mg/kg per day administered in divided doses either parenterally or orally for 10 days is usually adequate in both adults and children over 1 year. Chloramphenicol may be used in conjunction with either streptomycin or gentamicin.

Tetracyclines

The tetracyclines are bacteriostatic, and their use can lead to the development of complications. However, they are deemed suitable for use in uncomplicated cases. Tetracycline at a dose of up to 2 g/day in adults and 25–50 mg/kg per day in children over 9 years is recommended. Doxycycline may also be used at a dose of 200 mg/day in both adults and children over 9 years. As normal when using this class of drugs, a loading dose may be necessary. Tetracyclines can be used in addition to other agents.

Other antibiotics

Ciprofloxacin has been shown to be effective against *Y. pestis* in laboratory and animal studies. However this and other fluoroquinolones have not yet been used in human cases. Penicillins, cephalosporins and macrolides have been shown to be ineffective or of variable effect in the treatment of plague and they should not be used for this purpose.[18]

Prophylaxis

Healthcare workers or others who come into close contact with infected patients should receive prophylactic treatment. It may also be suitable for scientific fieldworkers investigating plague foci. Tetracycline, doxycycline or co-trimoxazole are currently used. Chloramphenicol has fallen from favour, due to the incidence of severe side-effects. Dosages used are: tetracycline 1–2 g/day in divided doses, doxycycline 100–200 mg/day and co-trimoxazole 1.6 g/day at 12-hourly intervals.[18]

Prevention

Vaccination is available; however, the likelihood of travellers contracting plague is very low. People going to work or live in areas where there is a known wild focus may be vaccinated. Laboratory workers who could be exposed to plague through clinical samples should be vaccinated in endemic areas, especially if investigating the focus. Development of immunity takes at least 1 month postimmunisation. Immunisation with the vaccine does not protect against developing primary pneumonic plague, so workers in risk areas, especially if geographically isolated, should be educated about signs and symptoms and encouraged to carry suitable antibiotics for immediate use if required. The vaccine is available through specialised centres, such as the Hospital for Tropical Diseases and the DoH. It is an unlicensed product, although if needed this is probably not significant.[19]

Avoiding exposure to rodents and their fleas, and controlling rodents and their fleas, remain the best methods of prevention. Domestic and companion animals in endemic areas should be treated for fleas, and bites and scratches avoided wherever possible.[20]

Rabies

(Hydrophobia)

In Chapter 1 it was stated that the UK benefits from certain geographic advantages in respect of zoonoses. Rabies is one of the most outstanding examples. The last indigenous case of rabies was in 1902, and after a nationwide campaign and enforcement of a system of strict quarantine the country was declared disease-free. The continued enforcement of these regulations and the strict rules relating to the issuing of pet passports has maintained the UK in this status; however, this is not true of continental Europe. The area where the disease is considered to be endemic advanced toward the coast of the English Channel at approximately 16 km (10 miles) each year during the last decade, and had engulfed Paris at one point. A massive concerted effort by the French government of vaccinating wildlife by using inoculated baits has led to the disease being pushed back towards the French border with other European states during the past 12 months.

During the last quarter of 2000 the WHO European rabies monitoring centre reported 1662 cases in Europe. Of these, 70% occurred in wild animals and 29% in domestic animals. There were only four human cases, all of which occurred in the Former Soviet Union.

Cases in domestic animals totalled 488, of which cats and dogs were the most significant pet species. Cases in cattle represent nearly half of the total, but onward transmission is unlikely. Bats are a significant reservoir for the disease in certain European countries; cases of bat rabies are usually only detected when they bite other animals or humans, therefore it is difficult to know the true incidence in the bat population. As the general public tends to associate rabies and dogs, it is advisable to remind individuals travelling to countries where the disease is endemic that bats and cats are also to be treated with caution, and to avoid contact with them if at all possible.

Most cases seen in European countries are designated as arising from 'fox-mediated rabies', where foxes are the main reservoir and vector. Other large and small mammals, including rodents, are less significant hosts.

Only Turkey has 'dog-mediated rabies', where wild and feral dogs form the main disease reservoir. The southern portion of the Former Soviet Union is unique in having a mixed pattern of dog- and fox-mediated infection.

European countries considered to be rabies-free are Albania, Finland, Greece, Iceland, Ireland, Italy, Macedonia, Norway, Portugal, Sweden, Switzerland and the UK and Northern Ireland. All other countries either have the disease or have had a case within the last 2 years.

Elsewhere in the world the disease is found in most countries and areas and some countries have high levels of disease incidence. These include areas of North, Central and South America, India, South-east Asia and Africa. In different geographical areas, different major animal reservoirs will be seen, linked to the most effective carnivore or scavenger species. Any other mammal in any country may become rabid, although not a primary vector or reservoir species. This said, canine rabies is considered to be the most significant animal reservoir worldwide.[21]

In 1996, the last year for which figures are available, over 33 000 human deaths from rabies were reported. The majority occurred in the countries forming the Indian subcontinent. The WHO suggests that there is significant underreporting of casualty figures, so the total death toll annually is well in excess of the figure given.

Approximately 50 million doses of various rabies vaccines are used in 10 million humans for postexposure treatments worldwide. No true figures are available for the incidence in China, although it is known that there is an extensive vaccination programme.

The expense of vaccine as postexposure prophylaxis for patients exposed to animals suffering from the disease or potentially rabid animals is a significant cost for the public health purse in countries or areas where the disease is endemic.

Rabies in the USA

Zoonoses are often seen as 'emerging diseases', either because the parameters of the relationship between humans and animals has altered in whatever way, or because a disease once believed to be controlled or eradicated has escaped from captivity and is on the rampage again. This is very true of rabies in the USA. Successfully controlled by vaccination and culling policies in domestic animals, new reservoirs of infection have now been identified in wild animal populations, from which infection claims human lives annually. Raccoons and bats are now the most significant animal reservoirs in the USA, while bat-borne rabies is seen as the most significant.[22]

The presence of a reservoir of disease in bats could almost be an excerpt from the script of a Hammer horror film. Bats are difficult to control, they are nocturnal, they are capable of living in large colonies in urban areas, and they are often protected by wildlife preservation statutes. The particular species of bat implicated in the 21 cases seen since 1980 is the silver-haired. This bat species has very sharp, small teeth and a bite could be small, unrecognisable and easily overlooked. In 20 of the 21 cases victims could not identify having been bitten or exposed to contact with a bat, although they or their families recalled bats being present in the patient's work place or home. This has led the US Centers for Disease Control and Prevention to issue guidance to clinicians that aggressive use of postexposure vaccination in individuals suspected of possible exposures to bats should be considered.[23]

The latest case in the UK

A man who contracted rabies after being bitten by a dog in the Philippines died in hospital in London on 8 May 2001. Hilario Laya, born in the Philippines but resident in the UK for several years, became ill after a trip to visit his family during which he was bitten by a dog. Mr Laya was admitted to the Hospital for Tropical Diseases in London on 30 April 2001 after he had started to show symptoms of rabies and was moved into isolation after admission to hospital. He was given a dose of rabies vaccine within an hour of being admitted and before a definite diagnosis was confirmed. On confirmation of the diagnosis he was sedated and moved into an intensive care bed. Sadly, treatment was started too late to alter the outcome.

This case highlights the need for travellers to be educated about this disease, and to realise that a bite from an animal requires medical attention as soon after it occurs as possible.

Disease in animals

The causative organism is a rhabdovirus, which is shed in large numbers into the saliva of infected mammals. Transmission follows inoculation of a bite wound or abrasion with infected saliva. Any animal suffering from rabies will display symptoms of central nervous system disturbance. After the incubation period and before the 'mad' or excitative phase, the animal may display certain prodromal symptoms. Behaviour will begin to change: animals may display antisocial behaviour becoming solitary, sexually aroused and having increased urinary frequency. The animal shows a lack of appetite for food and will not drink. After a few days the animal may become very excitable and vicious, biting or attacking anything or anybody in close proximity. This phase may be prolonged or short, and in some species it is totally absent. The third or paralytic stage of the disease follows. As paralysis sets in, the animal becomes progressively more docile and death follows rapidly, usually within 10 days of clinical signs beginning.

Transmission

Humans contract the disease from bites of rabid animals, or by inoculation of wounds with virus-containing saliva. The possibility of airborne droplet transmission has been demonstrated in caves where there are large populations of bats. The possibility of contracting the disease by corneal transplantation from patients dying of undiagnosed disease has also been documented.

Disease in humans

The virus is localised for a period postexposure in the immediate vicinity of the wound. The area around the site of entry may be painful or itch. Localised numbness, especially of the limb nearest the site, may be reported. There is a prepatent period following infection: this period seems to vary according to where the wound is in relation to the central nervous system. The closer the wound, the shorter the period; however, it is usually between 2 and 8 weeks, with variations linked to amount of inoculum and age of the patient – higher inocula and younger patients show more rapid onset of disease. Incubation periods of more than a year have occasionally been reported.

The virus migrates from the point of inoculation during this period, and enters the central nervous system. Early symptoms are very generalised, consisting of fever, headache and lassitude. As the central nervous system involvement begins, more serious clinical signs occur, often with acute onset. Symptoms progress as the neurological involvement increases. These can include insomnia, confusional states, anxiety, paralysis, hypersalivation, with swallowing difficulties caused by spasm of the oesophageal and laryngeal muscles (leading to the classic symptom of foaming at the mouth), altered perception and aggression. The patient may be extremely excited and often has convulsions. Disturbances of normal breathing and cardiac function are also seen. In the final stages of the disease most victims pass through phases of delirium, convulsions, and to almost invariable outcome of death.

The synonym of hydrophobia for the disease relates to the physical difficulties of drinking experienced by humans and animals, which are probably exacerbated by the abnormal mental state that occurs. The duration of the disease is short: death follows within a few days of clinical signs beginning.

Person-to-person transmission is extremely rare; however, precautions should be taken to prevent exposure to the saliva of the diseased person.

Diagnosis

Diagnosis is often presumptive from the patient's history or presence of bite wounds. The virus can be isolated from bodily fluids or tissue samples and identified by microscopy, after treatment with fluorescent antibody staining techniques. Rabies nucleic acid can also be detected using polymerase chain reaction tests. Isolating and identifying the virus from brain tissue or saliva postmortem often confirms diagnosis.

Treatment and prevention

Vigorous cleansing of bites or wounds with copious amounts of surfactant disinfectants or soap and water is a vital measure to reduce the risk of infection. This must be carried out immediately or as soon after the event as is practicable. In children, any bites are usually on the limbs, head, face or neck and they must be cleaned very thoroughly. Rapid use of postexposure vaccination is recommended.

Postexposure treatment also uses human rabies immunoglobulin (antirabies immunoglobulin) locally infiltrated around the wound site with concurrent administration intramuscularly. The dose used is calculated on a weight basis at a rate of 20 units/kg, split as 50% used locally and 50% intramuscularly. This is available in the UK from PHLS laboratories and regional blood transfusion centres in England and Wales. It is also available from Bio Products Laboratory and the Scottish National Blood Transfusion Service (addresses below).[24]

In patients with overt clinical signs intensive care is required to maintain respiration. If convulsions and seizures are controlled using anticonvulsants, there is a very small chance of survival.

The avoidance of bites and scratches from stray dogs or companion animals in countries where rabies is endemic is the most important part of any prevention strategy. Vaccination programmes in domestic animals, with rigid guidelines on the control of stray or feral dogs, cats and other mammals, are important in reducing risks and reducing exposure in countries where the disease is present. For island nations, rigid control of animal imports and the use of pet passport schemes or quarantine facilities allow their disease-free status to be maintained.

As has been previously mentioned, the vaccination of wild animal populations using inoculated baits has become very important in reducing levels of disease in the wild animal reservoir within endemic areas.

Travellers to rabies-endemic countries should be warned about the risk of acquiring rabies, although rabies vaccination is not a requirement for entry into any country. Pre-exposure rabies vaccination should be considered for patients who will be staying a month or more in countries where dog rabies is endemic. The necessity of postexposure rabies prophylaxis after an animal bite should be discussed with patients planning to travel to a non-industrialised country. They should be made aware that vaccination within a few days following a bite is capable of preventing the disease developing.

All travellers to such countries may wish to ensure that they carry sterile packs containing needles and syringes. In the event of needing vaccination, clean equipment will then be available. Travellers should be encouraged to avoid handling, feeding or caressing wild and feral animals unless wearing appropriate protective clothing.

Individuals at risk of occupational exposure, such as workers in laboratories, quarantine facilities, port officials, customs officers, animal and bat handlers and veterinary surgeons, whose employment is likely to carry a higher risk of exposure, should be considered for routine immunisation. Healthcare workers likely to be exposed to patients with the disease must be immunised wherever possible.

Vaccination regimes

There are wide regional variations in the types of rabies vaccines available. In the UK a human diploid cell rabies vaccine (HDCV: Pasteur Mérieux) is available, as is also a purified chick embryo cell (PCEC) vaccine (Rabipur: MASTA). In other countries, especially developing nations, other products may be in use. These include neural tissue vaccines prepared from sheep or mouse tissue. These vaccines have a high incidence of associated neurological complications; however, they may be the only product available. Some countries also use more modern vaccines prepared on different substrates to those in common use in western Europe or the USA. These include purified Vero cell rabies vaccine (PVRV), and purified duck embryo vaccine (PDEV).[25]

The DoH recommends that for prophylactic use HDCV vaccine should be given in a three-dose schedule on days 0, 7 and 28, with booster doses every 2–3 years if the individual is at continued risk. Where there is a short notice requirement for travellers, two doses given 4 weeks apart may be acceptable provided postexposure treatment is readily available. Booster doses should be given 6–12 months after the first dose, with subsequent doses every 2–3 years if required.

For individuals likely to travel to countries where there is a risk that postexposure therapy may be unavailable, or with products of dubious quality, a comprehensive pre-exposure programme is recommended. Although pre-exposure vaccination does not eliminate the need for additional therapy following an incident, it does simplify postexposure treatment by removing the need for rabies immunoglobulin and by decreasing the number of doses of vaccine required.

Where it is not known what regime (if any) a patient has been given as prophylaxis, a full postexposure regimen must be adopted unless there is serological evidence of antibody response.

Recommended postexposure regimens differ according to the previous vaccinations given. Fully immunised patients exposed to whatever level of risk should be given two booster doses on days 0 and 3–7. Individuals who have not been previously immunised, or who may have inadequate or out-of-date prophylaxis, should receive a course of injections starting as soon as practicable after exposure on days 0, 3, 7, 14 and 30 with a dose of rabies immunoglobulin on day 0.

Healthcare staff who have attended patients suspected of or actually suffering from rabies should be offered immunisation. Four doses of 0.1 ml HDCV at different sites intradermally on the same day have been suggested as adequate, provided the intradermal administration is carried out correctly. This regime is unlicensed.

Concomitant treatment with antimalarials, such as chloroquine and mefloquine, interferes with the antibody response to HDCV. For patients taking these medicines, intradermal vaccination is not recommended. The intramuscular route must always be used.

As with other immunisations, there may be a reaction to the injection. Pain can occur at the injection site, with reddening, swelling or itching. Headaches, nausea, gastrointestinal disturbance, generalised aching and dizziness have been reported. Due to the serious nature of the disease, postexposure programmes must be continued despite mild localised or systemic symptoms, or other factors such as pregnancy. The gluteal muscle must not be used as an administration site, as past experience has shown that there is a poor response to vaccine administered here.

WHO recommendations

The WHO endorses the use of the Essen regimen in postexposure vaccination. This consists of five injections of one dose of vaccine intramuscularly on days 0, 3, 7, 14 and 28. Day 0 is considered to be either the day of the injury or the date at which treatment begins. In theory both should coincide; however, in practice this may not always be the case. In addition to this vaccination scheme, three regimens have been developed to reduce the cost but not the effectiveness of postexposure treatment.

These are the 2.1.1 regimen, where two intramuscular doses of vaccine are given on day 1, and a single-dose booster on days 7 and 21. This scheme is particularly of value where there has been no physical damage, just exposure of skin or abrasions but not wounds to contamination by animal saliva.

The 2.2.2.0.1.1 regimen is for use with PVRV, PCEC vaccine or PDEV. It consists of intradermal injections of one-fifth of the intramuscular dose of vaccine – a dose dependent on the type of vaccine in use – at two sites on days 0, 3 and 7, and at one site on days 30 and 90.

The 8.0.4.0.1.1 regimen is recommended for use where HDCV and purified PCEC vaccine are available. The scheme consists of using a dose of 0.1 ml intradermally at eight different intradermal sites on day 0, four sites on day 7, and one site on days 28 and 90. This scheme is recommended by the WHO for severe exposure where there are single or multiple deep penetrating bites or scratches, or where contamination of mucous membranes with saliva has occurred and where no immuno-globulin is readily available.

As mentioned previously, part of the protection and prevention measures in place in the UK is a strict quarantine system. Recently this has undergone a slight modification to allow a pet passport scheme to be trialled. This section would not be complete without some details of the scheme.

Pet Travel Scheme (PETS)

This scheme was introduced in the UK in April 2000. The regulations, made under SI 1999 no. 3443 The Pet Travel Scheme (Pilot Arrange-ments) (England) Order 1999, form the basis of the scheme. It aims not only to prevent rabies entering the UK, but also to prevent establish-ment of *Echinococcus multilocularis* and certain tick-borne diseases endemic elsewhere in Europe and the rest of the world. It does not replace the quarantine system; however, it does allow cats and dogs, especially hearing dogs for the deaf or guide dogs for the blind, to accompany their owners abroad.

To enter an animal into the scheme, it must have a microchip inserted to identify it permanently, and be verifiably and effectively vac-cinated against rabies. A certificate is then issued under the scheme. This allows the animal to enter or leave the UK by specified routes and car-riers. Details can be found on the DEFRA website (http://maff.gov.uk/defra). Booster injections have to be given as recommended by the rabies vaccine manufacturer to maintain immunity and validity of the certificate.

In addition to this certificate, there is a requirement for the animal to be treated for ticks and tapeworms at least 24 hours before it enters or re-enters the UK. Again a certificate is issued by a vet to verify that the treatment has taken place with approved products on each occasion. These certificates must be obtained before travelling, otherwise the ani-mal may not be accepted by the travel company or may be turned back at the border.

Useful addresses

Bio Products Laboratory (BPL)
Dagger Lane
Elstree
Herts WD6 3BX
Tel: +44 (0)20 8905 1818

Scottish National Blood Transfusion Service (SNBTS)
Protein Fractionation Centre
Ellen's Glen Road
Edinburgh EH17 7QT
Tel: +44 (0)131 536 5700

References

1. Pearson G S. *The Threat of Deliberate Disease in the 21st Century*. In: Stimson Centre report no. 24. *Biological Proliferation: Reasons for Concern, Courses of Action*. Bradford: Stimson Centre for Peace Studies, Bradford University, 1998.
2. BBC News Online. Anthrax. http://news.bbc.co.uk (18 August 2000.)
3. Meselson M, Guillemin J, Hugh-Jones M, *et al*. The Sverdlovsk anthrax outbreak of 1979. *Science* 1994; 266: 1202–1207.
4. Jernigan J A, Stephens D S, Ashford D A, *et al*. Bioterrorism-related inhalational anthrax: the first 10 cases reported in the United States. *Emerg Infect Dis* 2001; 7: 1–26.
5. Lightfoot N F, Scott R J D, Turnbull P C B. Antimicrobial susceptibility of *Bacillus anthracis*. *Salisbury Med Bull* 1990; 68 (suppl.): 95–98.
6. Lederberg J. Infectious disease and biological weapons. Prophylaxis and mitigation. *JAMA* 1997; 278: 435–436.
7. Ingleby T V, Henderson D A, Bartlett J E, *et al*. Anthrax as a biological weapon: medical and public health management. *JAMA* 1999; 281: 1735–1745.
8. Mehta D K, ed. *British National Formulary*, vol. 42. London: British Medical Association/Royal Pharmaceutical Society of Great Britain, 2001.
9. World Health Organization. *Ebola Haemorrhagic Fever*. WHO fact sheet no. 103. Geneva: WHO, 2000.
10. Morvan J, Colyn M, Deubel V, Gounon P. *Ebola: virus marks detected in terrestrial small mammals*. Paris: Institut Pasteur, 2000.
11. World Health Organization. *Ebola Haemorrhagic Fever WHO Report*. Geneva: WHO, 2000.
12. *Uganda Ebola virus outbreak officially over*. Press release. Geneva: World Health Organization, 2001.
13. Bahmanyar M, Cavanaugh D C. *Plague Manual*. Geneva: WHO, 1976.
14. Dennis D T, Gage K L, Gratz N, *et al*. WHO *Plague Manual: Epidemiology, Distribution, Surveillance and Control*. Geneva: World Health Organization, 1999.

15. Galimand M, Guiyoule A N, Gerbaud G, *et al*. Multidrug resistance in *Yersinia pestis* mediated by a transferable plasmid. *N Engl J Med* 1997, 337: 677–680.

16. Chanteau S, Ratsifasoamanana L, Rasoamanana B, *et al*. Plague, a re-emerging disease in Madagascar. *Emerg Infect Dis* 1998; 4: 101–104.

17. Goddard J. Fleas and plague. *Infect Med* 1999; 16: 21–23.

18. Russell P, Eley S M, Green M, *et al*. Efficacy of doxycycline and ciprofloxacin against experimental *Yersinia pestis* infection. *J Antimicrob Chemother* 1998; 41: 301–305.

19. Anonymous. Prevention of plague. *MMWR* 1996; 45: 1–15.

20. Doll J M, Zeitz P S, Ettestad P, *et al*. Cat-transmitted fatal pneumonic plague in a person who travelled from Colorado to Arizona. *Am J Trop Med Hyg* 1994; 51: 109–114.

21. Fishbein D B, Robinson L E. Rabies. *N Engl J Med* 1993; 329: 1632–1638.

22. Noah D L, Drenzek C L, Smith J S, *et al*. Epidemiology of human rabies in the United States, 1980 to 1996. *Ann Intern Med* 1998; 128: 922–930.

23. Hoff G L, Mellon G F, Thomas M C, *et al*. Bats, cats, and rabies in an urban community. *South Med J* 1993; 86: 1115–1118.

24. Debbie J G, Trimarchi C V. Prophylaxis for suspected exposure to bat rabies. *Lancet* 1997; 350: 1790–1791.

25. Anonymous. Availability of new rabies vaccine for human use. *MMWR* 1998; 47: 18–19.

7

Emerging zoonoses

Healthcare is always changing. Not only do new products and new techniques affect practice, but there is also a continual challenge to the system from new disease states. The simplistic view that all mortality in human beings can be related to either the heart stopping beating and/or respiration ceasing is historically accurate. Without testing facilities or the techniques available to identify and classify the organism or condition responsible for death in an individual, misdiagnosis or a very general finding was often the only comment available for entry on the death certificate.

In the last 50 years, as we have looked deeper into the world of infection and pathogens, using better research resources and instruments, we have found more pathogens and identified more disease states. This holds true in the realm of zoonotic disease. The ability of a zoonosis to become of clinical importance does not solely rest on the ability of a pathogen to cross the species barrier, although this is a significant factor. The pathogen must have the opportunity to cross that barrier, and that is often related to other external factors. A change in the ecosystem, the meteorological pattern, global warming, farming practice or food handling can significantly alter the potential a known or unknown pathogen has to cause disease in humans.[1]

All of the disease states which have been discussed in this book so far are unquestionably zoonoses. Virtually everything about the disease is known, the pathogen is well recognised and usually detectable and classifiable, we understand the clinical course of the disease, the likely infective pathway and any treatment that is possible. For the conditions in this chapter, some or all of these parameters are not known. The conclusion that the disease is zoonotic may be made from detecting, culturing, and typing the causative organism in humans and beasts; however, the linkage between the two – being the transmission pathway or route – is either not well defined or purely theoretical. Treatment regimes may not be defined due to a lack of success with empirical treatment or the inability to identify a useful drug or treatment regime before either death or recovery intervenes.

Another factor that delineates the emergent pathogen is its ability to undergo gradual genetic modification, in a manner reminiscent of Darwin's finches, so that it reinvents itself as better adapted to exist in a particular population. This change can enable an organism which is benign in other species to become an efficient pathogen in humans or animals. Another factor is exposure: in many parts of the world forest clearance or the pressure on other habitats brings humans and animals into close encounters. Sometimes these will be species or populations which have previously remained apart. As we know from the introduction of smallpox into the Americas by the Spanish, the result of the exposure of previously discrete groups to the pathogens of others can produce devastating effects.

It is not only pathogens that can migrate: the trade in used tyres has successfully spread mosquitoes from one country to another in the stagnant water they may contain. Non-degradable plastic containers capable of holding rainwater make viable alternatives to traditional wetland habitats for mosquitoes to maintain breeding populations. A rise in the density of a vector population can allow a previously species-discrete pathogen with a zoonotic potential to break out of its normal niche.[2]

Luckily, in the UK we are unlikely to encounter this particular scenario. Our landscape has remained almost unchanged for centuries, and having eradicated all our major predator species and reduced other species to extinction, our opportunity to encounter an isolated population of another species with an associated reservoir of a major zoonotic pathogen is minimal. The unexpected can still happen when the safeguards of good practice or common sense are ignored. In terms of common sense, feeding dead sheep to cattle defies belief, and has led to unforeseen but nevertheless dramatic consequences. Apart from variant Creutzfeldt–Jakob disease (vCJD), which can be seen as an emerging pathogen or disease state, we are currently relatively safe within the UK, as far as our state of knowledge indicates.

Many emerging pathogens are seen in tropical and subtropical areas, either because the relationship of humans with animals is closer, or because environmental factors such as extreme heat encourage workers to be less careful as to their use of protective clothing. Another factor that affects the emergence of diseases is climate. High levels of ambient environmental heat and humidity allow pathogens to survive in the environment for longer and multiply faster on a susceptible host. Environmental change can also lead to new patterns of disease. West Nile virus (WNV) has displayed a formidable ability to alter its range, associated with changes in migratory bird patterns and the increase in suitable mosquito vector populations. It is of note that this particular disease requires both of these factors to be present in the same geographical location for it to become a threat. The presence of infected birds or suitable mosquitoes alone is not enough to precipitate an outbreak, thus giving us a chance to control the disease. It is only by careful study of the associated epidemiology of these diseases, their routes of infection and natural reservoir that we can gain the insights necessary to put in place the measures needed to prevent epidemic zoonoses outbreaks. In several of the zoonoses mentioned in this chapter, scientists involved in the outbreaks had to make informed assumptions from the case profiles or from the epidemiological pattern. Wherever these are of importance they are included in the text, as examples of the thought and deductive processes essential to disease management.

The following sections describe several pathogens, mostly viruses, that have shown zoonotic potential in the most dramatic manner by causing human illness, often with associated fatalities. The others are probably more spectres than reality, being fuelled by press reportage to the point where the smallest mouse roars like an enraged lion. The last section deals with zoonoses that are on the margins of scientific consciousness – the 'X-files' of disease. The diseases are either zoonotic or strongly suspected of being so; however, their potential or severity, and many of the other parameters of infection and pathogenesis, are unknown or untested. All of these ailments can be classified as emerging. It is impossible to predict how serious an outbreak would be, and what significance it would have for the human population.

In the context of the diseases explored in this section it is also worth considering that emerging infections or diseases may actually be re-emerging. Systems break down, and the reasons for public or personal health measures may become forgotten or lost in the mists of time. Several pathogens which were scourges of past ages are showing a resurgence, with outbreaks highlighting ageing or decaying infrastructure systems, such as sewage or water treatment, and the failure of consumers to know, understand or heed common-sense warnings related to animal handling or food preparation. It also worthy of note that the knowledge base of most healthcare practitioners does not extend beyond their years – we are children of our times. Symptoms and signs that would have sent alarm messages to our forebears leave us oblivious to the fate that may await. The lesson from the current outbreaks of human tuberculosis in the UK is that pathogens can only rarely be designated as eradicated; they are more likely to be in a state of abeyance, awaiting the chance to go on a rampage of infection.

The price of our continued safety in western Europe behind the ramparts of our healthcare and social systems is constant vigilance. Worldwide this role is borne by public organisations charged with the monitoring of public, human and animal health. In addition the World Health Organization (WHO) and other organisations such as the Institut Pasteur have networks of laboratories worldwide which undertake surveillance on a spectrum of diseases, some of zoonotic origin. Detection and identification are assisted by continual testing of indicator populations of susceptible species. In the USA the presence of WNV is monitored by just such a programme using regularly inspected captive domesticated birds to determine ambient levels of the causative organism. Similar to the canary in a cage in a submarine or mine, these precautions are designed to alert the experts and the populations for which they are responsible to the likelihood of an outbreak.

In the event of an outbreak of a zoonotic disease, there is a requirement for the lead organisation to be identified quickly and for it to take charge of all aspects of the outbreak. On occasions this is a difficult process, as rivalry and maintenance of jurisdiction often becomes more of an issue than the disease itself. It behoves anybody involved with an outbreak to remember that all other issues are peripheral to controlling the disease and preventing human casualties and fatalities.

Hendra virus

This pathogen was first identified after a respiratory tract illness was seen in 20 horses and two humans in Hendra (a suburb of Brisbane), Queensland, Australia, during September 1994. The resulting fatalities included 13 of the horses and one human. A second unconnected outbreak was identified as having occurred in Mackay, Queensland, in or about August 1994. The Mackay outbreak was much smaller – only two horses died and one human was infected, and later died. The outbreak was only identified retrospectively after the death of the man, 12 months after his exposure to infected horses. A third outbreak in January 1999, near Cairns, Queensland, killed only one horse.[3]

Initially the causative virus was named equine morbillivirus; this was later changed to Hendra, after the geographic site of the first documented outbreak. A paramyxovirus, closely related to measles and rinderpest, it had not been identified previously as responsible for disease in either humans or horses.

Disease in animals

In horses, the disease causes respiratory distress, fever, pulmonary oedema, and nasal and oral discharge with blood present. As the disease progresses, there is central nervous system involvement. Fruit bats with the virus have been found in Australia and Papua New Guinea. Experimentally the virus can cause severe disease in cats, which can pass viable organisms in their urine, as can horses. Horses could be infected by consuming feed contaminated with the virus, although the initial route of infection for any of the outbreaks is unknown.

Transmission

The route of transmission from horse to human initially seemed to be by contact with infected blood or secretions. Investigations since have shown the presence of the causative pathogen in fruit bats, which seem to form the normal reservoir in which no clinical signs of disease are seen.

Close contact seems to be sufficient for horse-to-horse spread; however, the route of transmission from bat to horse is as yet not elucidated. There has been no evidence of bat-to-human spread, or human-to-human spread in this disease.

Disease in humans

The virus is not deemed to be highly contagious; however, once clinical disease is seen the outcome is usually fatal.

Prevention

Good hygiene practice and quarantine of infected animals help control outbreaks.[4]

Nipah virus

In the period between late 1998 and mid 1999, there were cumulative reports of a novel form of encephalitis causing fatalities and neurological damage in pig workers in Malaysia. Three major clusters of cases were seen. The first was near Ipoh in the state of Perak, the second in Sikamat in Negri Sembilan, and the third and largest in Bukit Pelandock, also in Negri Sembilan.[5]

At first the disease was considered to be Japanese encephalitis. However, the pattern of infection, the scale of the outbreak and the predominance of mature male Chinese pig farm workers led to the conclusion that a zoonotic agent was implicated.

Transmission

A novel paramyxovirus related to but not identical with Hendra virus was identified as the causative organism. Most victims were of Chinese ethnicity – an important factor in determining the animal origin of the virus. In Malaysia, where there is a diverse ethnic mix, ethnic Malays are predominantly Islamic and are therefore not involved in the pig industry. No cases were seen in this group. If a widespread environmental vector such as a mosquito had carried the pathogen responsible for the disease, this distinct identification of victims by ethnicity and employment would not have been seen.[6]

Of the patients identified as suffering from the disease, 93% were involved in pig farming or associated activities. Of those patients with positive disease findings who were able to respond to questioning, the majority reported contact with swine before developing symptoms and a large proportion of these patients stated they had contact with pigs that were already ill. This evidence strongly indicated that pigs were the source of the disease. On the farms where human cases were seen, the pigs were also dying of a disease characterised by symptoms of respiratory tract infection and insufficiency. This led to the conclusion that the route of infection could be the inhalation of infected aerosols.

Disease in humans

The period between exposure to swine and overt disease was estimated to be usually less than 14 days from the histories taken from patients or their relatives. The main symptoms seen at the onset of clinical disease were neurological, with drowsiness and lowered levels of consciousness, loss of muscle tone, sensory and cerebral dysfunction, progressive disorientation, seizures, muscle spasm and spasticity. Generalised symptoms such as headache, dizziness and sickness were also seen in some cases, before or associated with the onset of more serious symptoms.

The disease progressed to encephalitis, with 32% of patients dying, 53% recovering fully, and 15% surviving but with persistent neural abnormalities and damage. In the Malaysian outbreak, of the 265 people affected, 105 died.

No human-to-human transmission has yet been documented, although familial clusters were seen. This probably relates to the pattern of employment on the pig farms, with whole families employed in the same enterprise. Healthcare workers who cared for patients suffering from Nipah virus or who were involved in their autopsies were all monitored for disease: none showed any clinical signs of contracting the condition.

Soldiers employed in the culling of pigs, abattoir workers and veterinary surgeons involved in outbreak control were also screened for antibodies to the virus.

Diagnosis

Confirmation of diagnosis was obtained by isolation of viral particles from the blood and cerebrospinal fluid of victims, both swine and human. In humans there were demonstrable abnormalities in both fluids. The viral particles, later genetically sequenced, were found to be identical in both pigs and humans, confirming the theory that the agent was zoonotic and had arisen in humans from initial swine infection.

Treatment

The only treatment available was generalised supportive therapy using aspirin and theophyllines. Half of the cases admitted to hospital lost consciousness and half of these patients required intubation and respiratory support. No intervention appeared to show any influence on the eventual mortality rate. On autopsy, damage was found in the central nervous system, lungs and kidneys. Using staining techniques, the virus was found to be present in neural and endothelial cells in the brain.

Prevention

It was decided that the main method of preventing further cases should be a comprehensive cull of all pigs in the Malay states of Negri Sembilan, Perak and Selangor. Approximately 890 000 pigs were slaughtered. Measures were put in place to prevent pig movements, to implement a health education programme, and to provide protective clothing and equipment to pig farmers. A system for national surveillance to identify and destroy any other herds identified as being infected was established. Following the cull, no new cases of the disease were seen.

In Singapore, by mid-March 1999, there were 11 cases of acute symptoms associated with the disease in abattoir workers reported to healthcare officials, of whom one subsequently died. All the infected individuals had handled imported pigs. A decision was swiftly taken to stop all imports of pigs from peninsular Malaysia and to close all abattoirs on 19 March 1999. Subsequent to these decisions no further cases were reported. Singapore has also banned racehorses and other horses from entering or returning from any of the constituent states of Malaysia.

Retrospective analysis of the infective pattern associated with the outbreak has led to the conclusion that the spread of the disease is related to the transportation of infected pigs, either from farm to farm, or from farm to abattoir. A dead dog was found to have the virus on autopsy; however, this was an isolated case. It is now believed that, in common with Hendra virus, the viral reservoir may well be fruit bats.

One of the less important but still significant effects of this outbreak is the lack of pork available for Chinese cookery, reducing the variety of dishes available in restaurants across the Malay peninsula.

Other unusual viruses in fruit bats

As a result of the emergence of Hendra virus, a research and investigation programme was set up to monitor diseases associated with fruit bats. Within the first 4 years two other viral diseases capable of zoonotic activity were identified in Australia.

In 1996 a virus related to rabies, now known as Australian bat lyssavirus, was found in a sick bat. A bat handler died after being infected with this pathogen in 1996 and in a separate incident in 1998 a further human fatality occurred.

Another paramyxovirus, now named Menangle virus after its first place of identification, caused an outbreak of disease at a piggery in New South Wales, Australia, in 1997. The pigs suffered illness, and sows spontaneously aborted. Human workers showed symptoms similar to influenza. Serological testing showed the virus to be the same in pigs and humans. The suspected reservoir is also fruit bats.

West Nile virus/Kunjin virus

WNV was first identified in the West Nile province of Uganda in 1937. A flavivirus, closely related to the causative pathogens of Japanese encephalitis and St Louis encephalitis, historically it has been confined to Africa, the Middle East and the Mediterranean coast. In the biggest outbreak recorded in 1974 in the Cape Province of South Africa, nearly 3000 humans were infected. Kunjin virus, which is very closely related and is believed to be a subtype of WNV, is found in Australasia and South-east Asia.

In Europe, WNV was first detected in Albania in 1958. The pathogen has since been detected in Portugal, France, Italy, Czech Republic, Slovakia, Hungary, Romania, Moldavia, Ukraine and Belarus. Most cases have coincided with periods of maximum activity for mosquitoes, usually July to September, when adjusted for the infectious prepatent period. Work in the USA has now demonstrated that the virus can over-winter in adult mosquitoes. Reintroduction into previously disease-free or quiescent areas may follow an influx of infected migrating birds.[7]

Disease in animals

The natural reservoir for the virus is wild birds. Especially significant is its presence in migratory species, as this forms a highly mobile infectious reservoir. Birds that become infected are believed to suffer from clinical symptoms of disease. As most are wild species, the course of infection is not easily determined although it is believed that the outcome is either death or survival. Birds that survive can become carriers.

The introduction of a carrier into a susceptible population of birds at a time when there is high seasonal mosquito activity can produce widespread infection, with a resulting 'die-off' of birds similar to that associated with the introduction of plague (*Yersinia pestis*) in susceptible rodents. Once the virus enters the mosquito population, it is also spread into any other mammals, including humans, which the insect bites. Transfer vertically through a generation of mosquitoes occurs by transfer from female adult to eggs laid postinfection. The other mammals usually affected include horses, bats, rodents, cats and raccoons.

Transmission

The disease is spread from bird to bird and from bird to human by a variety of mosquito species, depending on the geographical area involved (Figure 7.1). The spread of the disease into either local bird or human populations is solely dependent on the presence or absence of suitable vectors if infected or carrier birds are present. Much work has been done to identify the main species involved; however, the spectrum is so diverse that it is best to assume that all migratory birds under suitable conditions can suffer from or carry the pathogen.

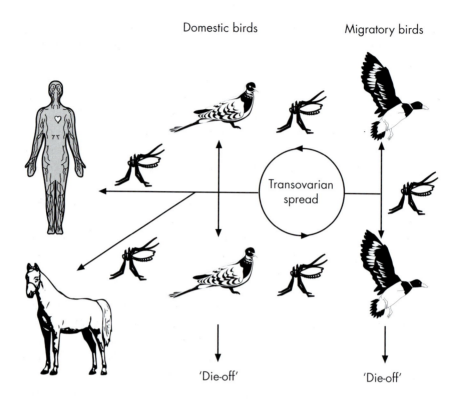

Domestic birds   Migratory birds

Transovarian spread

'Die-off'   'Die-off'

Figure 7.1 Cycle of infectivity and maintenance for West Nile virus in bird and vector populations.

Incidence

The most important outbreaks in the last decade were in Senegal in 1993, Romania in 1996, where out of 500 reported cases approximately 50 people died, Israel and Kenya in 1998, and Volgograd, Russia, in 1999 with 826 cases, of which 84 progressed to meningitis with approximately 40 fatalities. Cases have also been seen in the Camargue region of southern France, where an outbreak killed 20 partially feral horses in 2000, although no human cases were reported.[8]

Although endemic in certain areas of the world, the disease did not receive any particular media attention until August 1999 when an outbreak occurred affecting the eastern seaboard of the USA. Between August and October there were 62 human cases reported and confirmed, with seven deaths. The centre of the outbreak was in Queens, New York City, where a large 'die-off' of birds, particularly crows, was seen shortly before the first human cases. Many birds representing a wide variety of species in the Bronx Zoo also died. Once confirmed by serological testing, the outbreak was determined to be the first outbreak ever seen in the USA.[9]

This outbreak seems to have arisen as a result of the coincidence of a number of environmental changes. The mosquito population had increased markedly, partially due to prevalent climatic conditions during the previous year, and also as a result of the cessation of insecticide treatments on areas of standing water in public parks. The cases in humans coincided with the active feeding phase of the mosquito life cycle.

Subsequent to this outbreak the virus seems to have managed to establish a presence in the mosquito population, with a further outbreak in 2000. Eighteen cases, including one fatality, and one patient left in a permanent vegetative state, were seen in New York and New Jersey. The virus was detected in mosquitoes and birds before the cases occurred.

During 2000 the WNV Surveillance System, set up in response to the 1999 outbreak in the USA, demonstrated an increase in the geographic range of WNV activity. Surveillance included monitoring mosquitoes, sentinel chicken flocks, wild birds and potentially susceptible mammals (e.g. horses and humans). In 1999, WNV activity was detected in only four areas – Connecticut, Maryland, New Jersey and New York. There was a dramatic increase in the year 2000, with activity being detected in 12 areas (Connecticut, Delaware, Maryland, Massachusetts, New Hampshire, New Jersey, New York, North Carolina, Pennsylvania, Rhode Island, Vermont, Virginia), plus the District of Columbia in Canada. This increase in reporting may be due to enhanced capability and surveillance; however, seven areas also reported severe neurological WNV infections in humans, horses and/or other mammal species.

The disease was also identified in 65 horses across seven states, and in other small mammals, including bats, rats, cats and raccoons. One case was detected in a skunk. Mosquitoes with the disease were found in five states. Over 4000 dead birds from 76 species were reported across 12 states. Crows were the most numerous species reported.

Disease in humans

After an infective bite there is a short prepatent period of about 7–10 days, followed by generalised symptoms similar to influenza. There may also be a widespread rash, conjunctivitis, diarrhoea, localised lymph node swelling and respiratory difficulty – this seems to be related to the particular strain of WNV responsible. The acute phase of the disease follows swiftly, with stiffness of the neck, high fever, vomiting and headache. There may be onset of either meningitis or encephalitis, with fatality of more than 40% in cases where symptoms are severest and where onset is swiftest. Neurological symptoms of confusion, altered states of consciousness, tremor, convulsions and coma may be seen related to the onset and progress of central nervous system infection. The highest mortality is associated with cases in elderly patients.

On autopsy, findings include extensive tissue haemorrhage, cardiac damage and brain damage with cerebral oedema and neural degeneration.

Prevention

Dr Jeffrey Chang of the US Centers for Disease Control and Prevention has developed a vaccine to protect animals, especially horses, against WNV. The vaccination of susceptible feral or domesticated animals could reduce the infective reservoir and, coupled with mosquito control programmes, will drastically reduce transmission rates in endemic areas. It is hoped that a vaccine for human use may soon become available.

The states of the eastern seaboard of the USA have instituted a major programme of detection and monitoring aimed at reducing the impact of any further disease outbreaks. Seventeen states are involved plus New York City and the District of Columbia, Canada. The programme uses populations of tame birds which are monitored for the appearance of the virus during the period when the mosquitoes are actively feeding, and transmission is most likely.

All mass 'die-offs' are monitored and viral testing is carried out on recovered corpses as part of epidemic prediction routines. Birds entering the USA as planned imports for the pet trade must be tested for the virus before they are allowed past quarantine.

Attempts are also being made to reduce mosquito populations, using sterilised females, insecticides and other measures. People are encouraged to avoid bites wherever possible, using repellents, nets or screens to reduce the number of insects entering houses or other buildings.

Japanese encephalitis

Japanese encephalitis is an encephalitis caused by a virus of the Togviridae family, and is endemic in most rural areas of South-east Asia, especially China, Japan, North and South Korea, and the eastern areas of the Former Soviet Union.

Disease in animals

Pigs and some bird species act as the animal reservoir for the disease, usually in rural areas with extensive paddy field cultivation where the mosquito vectors can breed. The conditions for the disease are also able to exist on the fringes of urban centres, where there is waste or other land under development. The disease is seasonal, and the infective peak is usually seen between June and September when the mosquitoes are actively feeding, although this will vary from area to area depending upon the prevalent climatic conditions.

Transmission

Transmission to humans follows the bite of a previously infected mosquito.

Disease in humans

Most cases are subclinical and asymptomatic; however, in cases where clinical signs are seen there is a high incidence of mortality, with up to a third of patients dying. The clinical course begins with high fever, and neurological symptoms rapidly follow with altered perception, confusion and coma. Half of the patients who survive demonstrate long-term neural and psychiatric damage associated with neural loss.

In endemic areas, children and the elderly are at the greatest risk. Elderly patients have a high mortality, and children, although surviving the illness, display long-term sequelae. Travellers are unlikely to contract the disease if they are visiting solely urban centres, but there may be a risk of the disease if they are visiting rural areas or are likely to stay in an area for prolonged periods of time.

Treatment

Treatment is purely supportive.

Prevention

A vaccine is available and those persons considered to be at risk whilst visiting endemic areas should receive a programme of three injections at discrete intervals. Whilst travelling, wherever possible staying in air-conditioned accommodation or using a mosquito net is recommended, coupled with appropriate use of insecticides and repellents.

Other zoonotic viral encephalitises

Throughout the world there are a significant number of zoonotic viruses that cause human encephalitis; many of these conditions are caused by arboviruses. An arbovirus is defined as an arthropod-borne virus and is transferred from their animal reservoir to humans via biting insect vectors. The usual arthropods involved in transmission of the viral pathogen from one host to another are either mosquitoes or ticks, both soft- and hard-bodied. As demonstrated by WNV, many of the viruses can be vertically transmitted to the next generation through the eggs of an infected female arthropod.[10]

Many arboviruses are confined to tropical forests; however, as the mobility of human beings and other mammals has increased, it is possible for an infected individual to travel to almost any area of the world and then display the symptoms of disease. The arboviruses mentioned here are zoonotic. There are many others which appear to have only a human-to-human cycle and are therefore excluded from this section. Most arboviruses can be classified as either dengue-fever-like, or encephalitides. They can be further subdivided into mosquito- and tick-borne groups.

Mosquito-borne encephalitides include Lacrosse virus (USA), eastern (EEE) and western equine encephalitis (WEE: USA), St Louis encephalitis (USA and Canada) and Venezuelan equine encephalitis (Central and South America). Yellow fever caused by a flavivirus transmitted by the mosquito, *Aedes aegyptii*, is found in wild primates; however the main reservoir is considered to be the human population.

Of these diseases, and of the equine encephalitises, EEE is believed to be the most lethal, with a case fatality rate of nearly 60% in some outbreaks. Survivors are frequently left with persistent neurological damage, including epilepsy and focal damage in portions of brain tissue. EEE is an alphavirus and is transmitted by mosquitoes from its animal reservoir in horses to humans.

Lacrosse virus is normally found in small mammals such as squirrels and chipmunks, and is again transmitted by mosquito bite.

St Louis encephalitis is caused by a flavivirus. It is only seen in the Americas and has been isolated from northern Canada to southern

Argentina. The natural reservoirs are birds and bats, although the pathogen has also been isolated from horses and other mammals. The animals do not display any symptoms. In humans the disease develops following inoculation by infected mosquito bites. The prepatent period is between 4 days and 3 weeks and, as with many of the other arboviruses, symptoms commence with fever. Most cases do not progress to encephalitis, although this is possible, and fatalities have occurred.

Tick-borne encephalitides include the tick-borne encephalitis subgroup, consisting of central European tick-borne encephalitis, Russian spring–summer encephalitis, Louping ill and Powassan virus. Colorado tick fever is the only major dengue-like viral pathogen transmitted by ticks and is confined to the USA.[11]

Central European tick-borne encephalitis cases are seen over the same geographical range as its associated tick vectors. These may be hard- or soft-bodied, with *Ixodes* spp. predominating (see Tularaemia, pp. 121–126). The disease tends to be biphasic, with an influenza-like illness followed by the development of encephalitis a week later. The clinical course of the disease only leads to death in fewer than 5% of cases, with occasional serious neurological sequelae in survivors. Russian spring–summer encephalitis is more severe, with fatal outcomes in 25–30% of cases.

Louping ill is the only zoonotic disease of this type found in the British Isles and it causes sporadic infections, normally in hill sheep. Few human cases have been reported and the clinical presentation is normally mild.

Only 20 cases of Powassan virus have been reported, with half of the cases being fatal. Luckily, the tick which spreads the disease between the normal animal reservoir of rodents and their mammalian predators does not frequently bite humans.

Colorado tick fever has a small geographical range in northwestern America and western Canada, and only at an elevation of greater than 1200 m (4000 feet). Caused by an orbivirus, clinical disease is usually mild in humans and follows a tick bite from the *Dermacentor* spp. which parasitise small mammals. Encephalitis is rare, but can be fatal. As the course of the disease is often subclinical, it is difficult to determine how many cases occur annually.

There are no treatments for any of these conditions. Prevention of insect bites and the development of vaccines are the only methods available to reduce human infection rates. Once infected, the only therapeutic interventions are those necessary to prevent secondary opportunistic infections and generalised use of anticonvulsants or other agents, and nursing strategies for symptomatic support. Intracranial pressure can be reduced using infused mannitol. Nutritional support may be required for those patients in a persistent or prolonged coma. There is, as yet, no evidence that any of the available antiviral drugs is effective in these infections.

Non-arbovirus conditions

The following two conditions are included for completeness and, as with other emerging zoonoses, there are aspects of the conditions which have unusual characteristics.

Borna disease virus

Described more than 200 years ago in the town of Borna, Germany, this is a fatal neurological disease primarily of sheep and horses, caused by an RNA virus of the Mononegavirales order, family Bornaviridae. It is interesting that the Monenegavirales order contains the following viral families: flaviviruses (WNV, St Louis encephalitis, Japanese encephalitis), paramyxoviruses (Nipah, Hendra) and the rhabdoviruses (rabies).[12]

Borna disease is unusual in that it appears that the virus itself is not the cause of the symptoms seen – it is the immune response of the victim that causes the underlying damage that produces the characteristic symptoms.

Disease in animals

The disease occurs in animals in sporadic outbreaks, primarily in Germany. There is also antibody evidence of infection occurring in Israel, Japan, Iran and the USA in horses. In animals the disease is usually subclinical, although more virulent forms may arise and produce fatalities. It is also found in sheep, cattle, rabbits and some exotic species such as llamas and hippopotami. Rodents may possibly form a wild animal reservoir. It is currently not believed to be present in the UK; however, the Department for Environment, Food, and Rural Affairs (DEFRA) is undertaking monitoring of horses and sheep for the presence of this pathogen. The Public Health Laboratory Service (PHLS) is also taking an active interest in monitoring human cases of mental illness where other factors are suspected.[13]

Transmission

The virus is transmitted via nasal secretions, saliva or tears, either directly or by contamination of food or water. There is a prepatent period of approximately 4 weeks in horses with the disease presenting with non-specific symptoms usually of fever, loss of appetite, colic and constipation. This can progress to neurological symptoms with loss of coordination, muscle weakness, gait and posture abnormalities, repetitive movements, and paralysis as encephalitis develops. The virus invades the central nervous system by migrating from peripheral initial infection sites down neurons. The illness normally lasts for 1–3 weeks, and those horses displaying the central nervous system symptoms have up to 100% fatality. Survivors can relapse if stressed.

The disease occurs seasonally in spring and summer and, although this could indicate a possible spread by arthropod vectors, no vector has been identified in Europe, although it has been found in ticks in the Near East.

Disease in humans

There is a possible link with psychiatric illness in humans. The clinical course of infection in humans is not documented, although surveys of patients have demonstrated a correlation between psychiatric disease in humans and the serological evidence of Borna disease virus antibodies showing either active or recent infection. The relationship is most frequent in cases where gait or postural abnormalities are present. Some psychiatric patients who develop fatal meningoencephalitis have also been shown to be Borna disease virus-positive.[14]

Hanta virus and Hanta virus pulmonary syndrome

The first occasion on which Hanta virus was recognised as a cause of human fatality occurred in Hantaan, Republic of Korea, in 1978. A member of the Bunyaviridae viral family, several genotypes have been identified since. These viruses have been identified as the cause of outbreaks of disease since the 1930s across Eurasia. In 1993, a cluster of fatalities in south-western USA was attributable to a previously unknown genotype, now designated the Sin Nombre virus. Of 42 confirmed cases, 26 people died.

Rodents form the natural reservoir for these viruses, and the species of rodent is linked to geographical area and viral strain. Infected rodents do not show clinical symptoms of the disease. The virus has also been found in birds in Russia, and cats in China.

Transmission

Transmission usually follows inhalation of infected aerosols of rodent saliva, urine or faecal material. Cases have been reported following rodent bites or wound inoculation with infected material.

Disease in humans

Classic Hanta virus infection usually presents with renal involvement and haemorrhagic features. The variant associated with Sin Nombre virus is atypical, with fever; headache, diarrhoea, muscle pain and respiratory symptoms gradually worsen into acute respiratory distress.

Diagnosis

Diagnosis follows polymerase chain reaction testing of clinical samples. No human-to-human spread has been reported.[15]

Treatment

Treatment is purely supportive. Maintenance of organ function is central to any regime.

Prevention

Prevention poses some interesting problems. In most areas of the world rodent populations can be controlled. For certain areas of the USA, this poses a problem. In these areas the rodent hosts of the virus may also carry plague, and their demise may lead to their associated, possibly infected, fleas seeking alternative hosts and provoking a plague outbreak.

Lessons for the UK

Although as yet no cases of WNV have occurred in the UK, it is conceivable that the changes in climatic conditions, migration patterns and mosquito populations could lead to this or similar diseases causing an unforeseen outbreak in a similar manner to the eastern seaboard scenario. It is known that birds from areas where WNV is endemic do migrate to these islands, and the only factor mitigating against an outbreak is the current lack of a suitable vector. The lesson from the emergence of WNV in the USA is that constant vigilance is necessary.[13]

It was not until late in the 19th century that malaria was finally eradicated from this country, with historical evidence showing that clinical cases were commonplace in marshy areas of southern England and Ireland prior to this. The 'marsh ague' was apparently tertian or quartan malaria, and was widely reported in low-lying areas. Although malaria is not a zoonosis, the condition is indicative of an active mosquito population, capable of transmitting other pathogens.

An increase in rainfall, a change in environment, either by inundation of previously reclaimed low-lying land or other alteration by natural or human agency, could rapidly lead to suitable conditions where migratory animal host, capable arthropod vector and human populations coincide to produce an emergent epidemic. It is important that healthcare professionals have an understanding of the patterns of emerging disease. One of the more public aspects of healthcare that has become acutely apparent has been the recent resurgence of tuberculosis caused by *Mycobacterium tuberculosis* and the lack of symptom recognition of what had been a previously prevalent and then 'eradicated' disease. To this end there is a need for a population of healthcare professionals who are able to recognise, if only from book knowledge, the signs and symptoms of unusual disease states.

References

1.   Murphy F A. Emerging zoonoses. *Emerg Infect Dis* 1998; 4: 429–435.
2.   Reiter P, Sprenger D. The used tire trade: a mechanism for the worldwide dispersal of container breeding mosquitoes. *J Am Mosq Ctrl Assoc* 1987; 3: 494–501.
3.   Selvey L A, Wells R M, McCormack J G, *et al*. Infection of humans and horses by a newly described morbillivirus. *Med J Aust* 1995; 162: 642–645.
4.   Williamson M M, Hooper P T, Selleck P W, *et al*. Transmission studies of Hendra virus (equine morbillivirus) in fruit bats, horses and cats. *Aust Vet J* 1998; 76: 813–818.
5.   Anon. Outbreak of Hendra-like virus – Malaysia and Singapore, 1998–1999. *MMWR* 1999; 48: 265–269.
6.   Goh K J, Tan C T, Chew N K, *et al*. Clinical features of Nipah virus encephalitis among pig farmers in Malaysia. *N Engl J Med* 2000; 342: 1229–1235.
7.   Hubálek Z, Halouzka J. West Nile fever – a reemerging mosquito-borne viral disease in Europe. *Emerg Infect Dis* 1999; 5: 643–650.

8. Tsai T F, Popovici F, Cernescu C, *et al.* West Nile encephalitis epidemic in southeastern Romania. *Lancet* 1998; 352: 767–771.

9. Asnis D S, Conetta R, Texeira A A, *et al.* The West Nile virus outbreak of 1999 in New York: the Flushing Hospital experience. *Clin Infect Dis* 2000; 30: 413–418.

10. Gubler D J. Resurgent vector-borne diseases as a global health problem. *Emerg Infect Dis* 1998; 4: 442–450.

11. Goddard J. Viruses transmitted by ticks. *Infect Med* 1997; 14: 859–861.

12. Richt J A, Pfeuffer I, Christ M, *et al.* Borna disease virus infection in animals and humans. *Emerg Infect Dis* 1997; 3: 343–352.

13. Meah M N, Lewis G A. *A Review of Veterinary Surveillance in England and Wales with Special Reference to Work Supported by the Ministry of Agriculture, Fisheries and Food 1999.* London: MAFF, 2000.

14. Herzog S, Pfeuffer I, Haberzettl K, *et al.* Molecular characterization of Borna disease virus from naturally infected animals and possible links to human disorders. *Arch Virol* 1997; 13 (suppl.).

15. Hughes J M, Peters C J, Cohen M L, *et al.* Hantavirus pulmonary syndrome: an emerging infectious disease. *Science* 1993; 262: 850–851.

8

Implications for healthcare

The other chapters in this book have aimed to explain the mechanics of zoonotic infection. This chapter aims to explore why as healthcare professionals we should use our understanding of these infections to identify and treat these conditions and offer advice on prevention strategies to our patients.

Significance of zoonotic disease

Although some of the zoonotic diseases in this volume are not dramatically significant in daily practice, there are others that cause serious disease, or whose prevention complicates the management of severely or chronically ill patients. The estimate from the Health and Safety Executive (HSE) of 20 000 episodes of zoonotic disease in agricultural workers in the year 2000 is not insignificant when viewed in terms of economic loss or personal misery.[1]

Zoonoses carry with them a cost, not just in purely monetary terms, and many of them are preventable. It is therefore important that whenever possible strategies are implemented to treat appropriately or prevent these diseases in order to safeguard scarce resources and thereby benefit patients.

One of the key objectives in writing this book was to provide a knowledge base to assist assessment of patients seen in primary care pharmacies. Information informs and shapes all healthcare practice, and knowledge of these conditions forms a part of the body of skills necessary in primary care. The practice of pharmacy is changing and there is an increased emphasis on a team approach to dealing with patients. The numbers of patients attending a pharmacy as their first point of contact with healthcare services is greater than ever before, and the skills and knowledge needed to signpost these patients accurately so that they obtain the best, most appropriate treatment for their conditions is also changing. There is a growing need for practitioners to obtain the widest skills and knowledge base possible to benefit both patients and colleagues.

The majority of zoonoses are untreatable at community pharmacy level, or at other first-contact sites such as NHS Direct. Nor do the healthcare professionals involved at these first-contact sites have the right of diagnosis and, at present, prescribing rights necessary to treat these conditions effectively. Therefore, after an oral history has been taken or physical symptoms have been noted, all patients who are suspected of being victims of these conditions should be referred to a medical practitioner as soon as possible. It may well be of benefit to write a referral note, especially where there is suspicion of a serious condition, so that the information and observations can be communicated to the medical practitioner. This is especially essential where there may be a period of time between the patient's presentation and the next available appointment at the doctor's surgery, or where it is possible that the symptoms displayed may be transitory, for example in the tick bites or tick attachment and erythema associated with Lyme disease.

Pharmacists and other healthcare professionals who undertake domiciliary visiting or have regular contact with patients over a prolonged period of time will often have an extensive knowledge not only of the patient but also of his or her domestic situation. This can be a key to understanding either a chronic or an acute exacerbation of a patient's condition, in which a zoonotic disease derived from a companion animal, work or immediate environment may be responsible. There is also an increasing call for health information and activity relating to either health improvement or prevention of illness. For at-risk patients with chronic conditions or who are on continual therapies, a requirement to initiate or enable a risk- or harm-reduction programme is desirable if not yet mandatory.[2]

Disease prevention strategies

There is a body of literature, much of it recently written, in relation to risk–benefit analysis in health issues. Zoonotic disease falls readily into this framework. Many of the risks have already been covered in some detail, so to set the scene for the rest of this chapter it is necessary to consider the benefits associated with animals in a social and domestic context.[3, 4]

Benefits of companion animal ownership

Most cat owners, when asked, state that they keep cats for companionship and affection. This group is not alone: other groups of companion animal owners will express similar sentiments, even if their companion animal of choice is a reptile or other creature which is perhaps less cuddly or less demonstrative.

Studies undertaken across the world have shown that the bereaved, the socially deprived, mentally ill and house-bound all exhibit lower symptom levels or improvements in their condition if they have contact with a companion animal. Reductions in blood pressure and improved recovery rates have been demonstrated in male subjects in one study.[5] The charity Pets as Therapy (PAT), which takes dogs into residential homes and other long-term care settings, justifiably claims to improve the quality of life of many patients.[5]

Children and adults who have behavioural difficulties or psychiatric conditions have been shown to improve if they have to care for another creature which in return demonstrates affection for them. The evidence appears to be convincing that the benefits are real, and not imagined, with far-reaching implications.[6, 7]

These benefits may come at a price, as there may be a risk to a patient from contracting a zoonotic disease. The next part of the process is the risk assessment and, if appropriate, implementation of a harm-reduction strategy.[8]

The next sections and the assessment process are focused on the already unwell or at-risk patient. It must be remembered that nobody is completely safe, and that individuals who are on their gap year, off to far-flung places to do voluntary service overseas, or outdoor pursuits, may require some health advice, although a full risk assessment and harm-reduction programme are usually inappropriate.

Benefits from domesticated animals

There is another aspect to be considered before passing on to the assessment stage. Domesticated and agricultural and other animals also have a societal role. Traditionally, animals have been kept for their products, be they eggs, meat, milk and milk products, hides for leather, wool or a wide variety of by-products such as gelatin, glycerin, hair or fats and oils. Although the number has reduced markedly over past decades due to social changes and higher costs, there are also individuals who work with wild or part-domesticated animals, such as pheasant and other game birds or deer, kept solely for hunting.

In social terms, a large number of people derive their employment from involvement in the rearing, husbandry, harvesting and processing of animals and their products. As in many other areas of human endeavour, the reward does not come without a risk. Employment in this industry carries with it an enhanced risk from certain pathogens, including some zoonoses. Individuals who have other predisposing factors which make them more susceptible to contracting disease may have some difficult choices to make if reducing their risk involves losing the benefit of continued employment.[9]

There are also a number of occupations where exposure to animals is part of the daily routine, but where exposure might be less obvious. Dog wardens, animal rescue workers, roofers, especially when working on roofs where pigeons or other birds have roosted, zoo and circus employees all stand at a greater risk of exposure to zoonotic pathogens than members of the general public.

Risk assessment

In both primary and secondary care settings healthcare workers often gain knowledge relating not only to the medication and/or physical condition of their patients, but also sometimes to their domestic situation, especially when domiciliary visits are undertaken. The presence of a companion animal and a basic knowledge of the likely zoonotic conditions associated with that species might assist in assessing the patient's risk.[10]

Recently a doctor told me that another partner in the practice had been treating an elderly woman for a prolonged period for a recurrent chest infection and persistent dry cough. A home visit had to be made after the woman had become acutely ill and an emergency call had been made. On examination, the woman was found to have a severe pulmonary infection again. It was only as the doctor prepared to leave that the elderly woman said that her cockatoo had been off-colour for a while, and that the vet was now treating it for its wheeze. Serological tests showed the lady to be suffering from psittacosis, and the condition resolved on prolonged antibiotic therapy.

This story has many lessons to teach. The moral for all healthcare workers is that it is essential, especially when carrying out a risk assessment, to have a comprehensive knowledge of patients and their lifestyle and circumstances. It is necessary to concentrate not just on the disease state, or more cynically, on the individual as a body with an interesting condition attached.

Accurate observations, asking the right questions and building a picture of the patient's condition are skills that all healthcare workers should develop. There must also be some knowledge of the likely pathogens associated with particular animals and the patient's circumstances.

A risk assessment for other reasons may form part of a patient's discharge procedure from secondary care, and it is essential for the risk of zoonotic disease to be included in an appropriate manner for certain patients. When a patient's history is being taken formally or during less formal procedures, any mention of a close association with animals should raise the issue, if only in the mind of the healthcare worker concerned.

To recap, the main identifiable risk groups are children, pregnant women, the immunocompromised patient, agricultural and food-industry workers, and the elderly or infirm. The main diseases associated with these groups are summarised in Table 8.1.

Having identified the animals the patient comes into regular contact with, a review of the possible disease states related to the animal is needed. Detailed information on these diseases can be obtained from the appropriate sections in previous chapters. Listing the diseases can help identify insertion points for control measures to stop transmission or reduce pathogen burdens.

When carrying out an assessment, it is important to remember that it appears that the absolute risk of contracting a zoonotic infection is dependent on additive risk factors. Children on farms, immunocompromised agricultural workers and pregnant food-industry operatives have a greater risk than a similar individual who does not have the additional risk factor. Absolute risk is also dependent upon other factors. Factors such as regular consumption of unpasteurised dairy products, frequent close contact with animals or poor personal hygiene practice add a further layer of risk.

It should be remembered that patients whose immune symptom is compromised or inadequate might not be solely those individuals suffering from human immunodeficiency virus/acquired immunodeficiency syndrome (HIV/AIDS). This category also applies to patients who are alcoholic, especially if cirrhosis is present; individuals with certain neoplastic diseases where chemotherapy, radiotherapy or high levels of steroids are being used; patients with renal, hepatic or splenic failure; diabetics; individuals suffering from certain congenital conditions including cystic fibrosis; sufferers from autoimmune conditions such as systemic lupus erythematosus where immunosuppressant therapy may be used; organ transplant recipients with concomitant immunosuppressant therapy; people who are malnourished; and haemodialysis patients. Patients on high-dose steroids or receiving long-term low-dose steroid therapy also show some loss of immunocompetence. The side-effects of such therapy pose a risk to the patient from many pathogens, and from

Table 8.1 Summary of diseases by risk group

Risk group	Main disease threat
Animal handlers	Leptospirosis *Pasteurella* Rabies *Salmonella* Tetanus
Neonates and children	Cutaneous larva migrans *Escherichia coli* Hookworm *Salmonella* Scabies Tetanus *Toxocara* Toxoplasmosis
Elderly and infirm	*Escherichia coli* Influenza *Listeria* Psittacosis *Salmonella* Tetanus
Agricultural and food-industry workers	Anthrax Brucellosis *Echinococcus* *Escherichia coli* Leptospirosis Orf *Pasteurella* Q fever *Salmonella* Tetanus Tuberculosis (*bovis*)
Immunosuppressed or immunocompromised individuals	*Campylobacter* Cat scratch disease Cryptococcosis Cryptosporidia *Escherichia coli* *Listeria* *Mycobacterium avium* complex Psittacosis *Salmonella* *Toxocara* Toxoplasmosis Tuberculosis (*bovis*)
Pregnant women	Gestational psittacosis *Listeria* *Salmonella* *Toxocara* Toxoplasmosis

physical damage that may lead to infection. Zoonoses are not the only risk to these patients; however, they should not be ignored.[11]

In essence, an elderly, immunocompromised agricultural worker who keeps pet cats in the kitchen, sleeps with the dogs, does not wash and regularly consumes pints of unpasteurised milk is either lucky, or dead.

Harm reduction and prevention

The gold standard for all healthcare has always been preventing a condition from establishing so that therapeutic intervention in clinically advanced symptomatic disease is rendered unnecessary. In zoonotic infection the old adage that 'Ten parts of prevention are better than one part of cure' holds very true. Once contracted there are certain zoonoses that are impossible or extremely difficult to eradicate. *Toxocara*, toxoplasmosis, tuberculosis and psittacosis all pose immense problems in ensuring that a sufferer does not relapse with a further attack after a course of therapy. In some individuals continuous or periodic treatment may be necessary to maintain a cure.[8]

However prevention, with the implied complete protection it offers, may be unachievable for a variety of reasons, and often the best that can be attained is a diminution of risk or a reduction in the harm that an infection may cause. For identified risk groups reducing the risk of contracting zoonotic infections forms an important part of the healthcare professional's role. The usual premise for harm reduction is that an attempt must be made to maintain patients' health, whilst seeking to least alter their overall quality and style of life the least. Realistically, to achieve this end, there is a need for patients to receive as much education and information relating to the risks they face, and the means of reducing those risks from exposure to zoonotic agents. This can be as simple as promptly cleaning up the cat litter tray, or getting somebody who does not have any predisposing condition to empty the tray for them. The information provided has to be geared to the patient's comprehension and there may be a corresponding need for counselling or support.

The main plank of any strategy is prevention of exposure or reduction of risk associated with exposure to a pathogen (Figure 8.1). Achieving this in patients who are already ill can be extremely difficult, as there often is a need to change long-standing habits, whilst trying to hold relationships, employment and private life together. This can be particularly difficult for patients where their condition is unlikely to

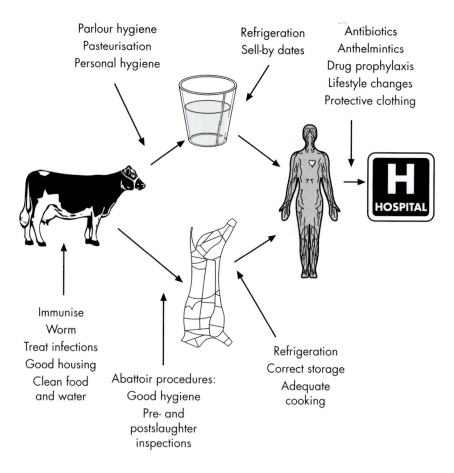

Figure 8.1 Prevention points and strategies for food-borne zoonoses.

improve, especially if one of their main sources of emotional comfort is a companion animal, rather than relatives or friends. Harm reduction becomes much less easy in patients who may have an occupational exposure to zoonotic pathogens.

With the current economic downturn and other difficulties that agricultural enterprises face, the last straw may be the loss of a worker, especially in a small operation. The effects for an individual can also be catastrophic, with loss of income leading to far-reaching lifestyle changes.[12]

It is essential that any part of an overall strategy or measure that can be achieved is a bonus. However resistant the patient may be, and however ill, there is usually something that can be done to reduce risk.

In a chronically ill patient, measures may have to be introduced gradually over long periods. The full spectrum of applicable measures may only be attained as the patient becomes comfortable with the necessary changes.

It is also essential that this be viewed as a multidisciplinary issue. The traditional core team in community care is expanding under the National Health Service reforms. Issues relating to zoonotic infection may cross the boundaries of social work, veterinary care, nursing, pharmacy and medical services. If one practitioner identifies an issue, then communication to other parties is essential. This becomes particularly true when dealing with patients whose condition may be chronic, and who require a large alteration to their lifestyle for risk reduction. The involvement of a vet, employment service advisors or benefit agency personnel – all classes of professionals not traditionally seen as healthcare workers – may be indispensable.[11]

Constituent measures for prevention strategies

Having identified what appear to be the main risk pathogens, the next step is to develop the components for a successful strategy. Table 8.2 provides a summary of the threat posed from a method of transmission, the mode of infection and the prevention measures that may be appropriate.

The framework shown in Table 8.2 can be used to assemble a list of possible measures which can be used to reduce transmission and infective risk. It is only a starting point. Most of the measures listed are voluntary; there is no legislation which forces companion animal owners to adopt any or all of the recommendations.

This is not true for workers in the agricultural or food industries, or in any other occupation where contact with animals or their products forms part of the normal work routine. Persons employed in this way have a greater duration and frequency of contact with animals, and therefore an increased likelihood of being exposed to zoonotic pathogens. The protective measures recommended for this group are already enshrined either in statute or in best custom or practice within the associated industry, usually under provisions of the Health and Safety at Work (HASAW) etc. Act, or the Control of Substances Hazardous to Health (COSHH) regulations. These are explored under the legislation section at the end of this chapter.[1]

There is also a risk group that falls between the companion animal owner and the commercial extremes. These are people who are employed as animal keepers in zoos and circuses and also the workers in

Table 8.2 Summary of prevention measures

Mode of transmission	Prevention measures
Pica/faecal contamination of food, water, clothing or skin	Education and personal hygiene Anthelmintics or antibiotics for animals and humans Prompt removal of faecal matter Disinfection of contaminated areas or items Thorough cleaning and cooking of food Ensuring water is clean by filtration or chlorination
Aerosol	Use of face masks (personal protective equipment or PPE)
Saliva	Avoid animal bites and disinfect wounds promptly Vaccinate animals and humans Avoid direct contact with animal's face Muzzle aggressive animals Educate owners not to kiss their pets
Blood	Cover open wounds
Vector-mediated	Use repellents Control life cycle at breeding sites Use insecticides/parasiticides Wear suitable clothing
Fomites contact	Clean surroundings thoroughly, and disinfect as appropriate Wear suitable protective clothing whilst undertaking risk activities
Food	Cook meat and eggs thoroughly Consume pasteurised milk and cheese Wash or clean food thoroughly Refrigerate items correctly. Do not consume past 'best before' or out-of-date items Use common sense and practise personal hygiene
In chronic or extreme cases	Consider drastic changes to lifestyle, including: • Changing employment • Avoiding contact with animals • Permanent removal of animals from domestic environment by rehoming or euthanasia • Controlling feral or pest animals in vicinity • Sterilising foodstuffs

protection societies and animal refuges or rescue centres, who may be volunteers or casual workers. There is a possibility that they can fall outside the scope of regulatory protection. Best practice would be for these individuals to adopt the measures required in industry; however, this may not be possible. For this group a mix-and-match approach to prevention measures is probably best. Where any doubt exists as to the hazards associated with a particular animal or procedure it is best to err on the side of caution.

So far the focus of this chapter has been upon the patient who is already unwell. What of the worried well or the population in general?

Health promotion and education

Healthy pets mean healthy people and vice versa. In general a companion animal which is regularly wormed, properly fed and bedded down will be less likely to harbour infection. The control of ectoparasites, regular veterinary care and domestic hygiene routines with the use of disinfectants, wearing protective gloves when handling faecal matter and preventing the animal biting, licking or scratching any human goes a long way to reducing accidental infection rates.[13]

As a prevention measure, the early education of children about the care of animals and good personal hygiene is important in preventing not only immediate disease, but also the establishment of an infective focus (such as toxoplasmosis) which, once contracted, may recur at a later juncture. General advice is usually available from veterinary surgeons and bodies such as the Pet Health Council that provides information leaflets and advice.

The information relating to prevention measures for patients, their carers, friends and relatives or healthcare professionals is also not difficult to access. As in many other fields of medicine, the USA has already produced a great body of work on these issues which is often overwhelming in its quantity, if not its quality. Some of the web addresses in Appendix 1 provide suitable starting points.

As with most medical conditions, many self-help groups are able to provide literature for use in patient education on the risk of zoonotic diseases and the appropriate management of companion animals either to prevent these diseases or to develop harm-reduction strategies.

This is an important field of health promotion where healthcare professionals are well placed to be effective advocates for both patients and their pets. There is a profound need for the void between veterinary care and traditional general-practitioner-led community services, where there may be little linkage between the pet and the patient, to be bridged. The problem of health education relating to zoonotic disease is an issue that must be grasped to protect the health of all owners of companion animals.

Healthcare professionals not belonging to the medical profession, and especially pharmacists, should consider rapid referral of any patient suspected of having a zoonotic condition to a doctor as soon as is practicable, as most of these conditions will not respond to self-medication.

Treatment

If the disease cannot be prevented, or the risk-reduction strategy fails, then the next option is treatment. This is usually with a therapeutic agent, be it an antibiotic, antifungal, anthelmintic or insecticide, though in some conditions (for example, hydatid disease) surgical intervention may also be necessary.

Resistance, especially in antimicrobial treatment, affects the effectiveness of any drug therapy, and this is becoming an increasing concern. Extensive studies are being undertaken by the Department for Environment, Food, and Rural Affairs (DEFRA, previously the Ministry of Agriculture, Fisheries, and Food or MAFF) and the Department of Health (DoH) in the UK with input from the Public Health Laboratory Service (PHLS) to ascertain the extent and significance of the problem. The World Health Organization (WHO) has issued guidelines on prescribing and supplying antibiotics and is also carrying out investigations of its own. The issue is significant when related to zoonoses, as animals are treated with the same antibiotics as humans. Any resistance developing in the animal population can spread into the food chain and thus affect the usefulness of these agents. The display of resistance to certain insecticides and anthelmintics should also be borne in mind when choosing an agent, and monitoring may be necessary to determine the chosen drug's efficacy.[14]

Many cases of zoonotic infection will never reach the stage of symptomatic disease, or be diagnosed, and are resolved by empirical general antibiotic treatment by a patient's general practitioner before full-blown clinical symptoms can manifest. More cases may be seen of certain diseases as blind use of wide-spectrum antibiotics declines.

In many cases of infection where a zoonotic disease is suspected, the rapid use of antibiotics is often imperative. Susceptibility testing may be necessary. Broad-spectrum blind usage, although not desirable, can be the fastest method to prevent progression. Combination therapies or progression to 'reserved' moieties may be necessary, especially if the course of the disease is rapid or morbidity is feared, although this normally requires diagnosis using appropriate measures.

Certain infections may require extended antibiotic therapy with the concomitant problems associated with interactions and choice of a suitable agent for sustained use. In immunocompromised patients there will be a requirement for specialist support in choosing, monitoring and supplying some drugs required for eradication or control of certain organisms, especially resistant strains of tuberculosis and *Cryptosporidium*. There may also be a need to keep latent infection suppressed for a patient's lifetime, as in toxoplasmosis, so expert advice is essential.

When choosing anthelmintics for worm infestations, the more unusual parasites may require drugs which are not in routine use and/or available on a named-patient basis only. In these cases support from specialised units can be invaluable. IDIS Ltd can provide many of these specialised drugs (see below for details).

The use of unlicensed products is a thorny issue, and the initiation of such drugs at primary care level may pose a serious clinical dilemma. It may be necessary to refer a patient to another healthcare provider, if practicable. In cases of more unusual organisms, especially if the condition has been contracted abroad, the Hospital for Tropical Diseases is usually the best informed, and best placed to undertake treatment. Its address and contact telephone numbers may be found at the end of this chapter.

General supportive therapies may also be needed for symptom control. The use of anti-inflammatories, painkillers, rehydration therapy or antinauseants may be appropriate. In specific conditions, i.e. hydatid disease, surgery may be necessary, requiring unusual drugs or adjuncts depending upon the severity or extent of infection, the organism responsible and the stage in its life cycle. Specialist support can again be invaluable.

The choice of pesticide in arthropod infestations needs to be carefully considered to ensure no underlying medical conditions are exacerbated. Press coverage of Gulf War syndrome has heightened public fear of pesticide use, but not in a balanced way. This has led to unreasoning fear of all insecticides. On that basis it is necessary not only to be careful in choosing an agent which will eliminate the arthropod concerned, but also which will not cause or increase the anxiety of patients or their carers.

Hypersensitivity to organophosphates and the emergence of resistant strains of arthropods are matters of concern, and influence the choice of agent. The formulation may also be important; the use of alcohol-based lotions or solutions is contraindicated in asthmatics.

Wherever possible, detailed information on treatments has been given in the appropriate single-disease sections. However, not all of these therapies are approved in the UK, so treatment must follow local or national policies or guidelines. The overriding authority is either the *British National Formulary* or local formularies when therapeutic choices are to be made, unless the condition is so unusual as to require empirical treatment.

Antimicrobial resistance

The ability of microorganisms to adapt to any conditions and challenges is remarkable. Their ability to develop resistance to currently available antibiotics has become of increasing concern. The emergence of methicillin-resistant *Staphylococcus aureus* (MRSA) and other organisms with multiple resistance to whole classes of antibiotics threatens to return the management strategies for certain diseases to the pre-penicillin era.

Concerns are frequently expressed over the use of antibiotics in animal feed and management programmes. In July 1998 a comprehensive review of the issues and data related to antibiotic resistance in the food chain was undertaken by the then MAFF. The House of Lords Select Committee on Science and Technology reported on resistance to antibiotics and other antimicrobial agents in 1998.[15] This highlighted the threat to human health, and a report *The Path of Least Resistance* from the Standing Medical Advisory Committee,[16] as well as recommendations made in the UK Antimicrobial Resistance Strategy and Action Plan produced by the National Health Service Executive in June 2000 have led to health authorities being required to develop local prescribing guidelines.

From the research available, it would appear that resistance to antibiotics in animal pathogens which may be zoonotic is selected following the introduction of veterinary medicines or growth promoters. This produces bacteria capable of being transmitted to humans by food; these bacteria are resistant to related human antimicrobial moieties. This can then lead to difficulties in successfully treating any disease thus caused. The use of antibiotics in agriculture is of particular concern in zoonotic disease, as the pathogens, by definition, are from animal sources.

The issue is not trivial, as some of the organisms in which resistance has been identified are not resistant to solely one antibiotic class but exhibit resistance across a range of antimicrobial groups.

Multiantibiotic-resistant pathogens of particular concern are those resistant to fluorinated quinolones (*Salmonella* and *Campylobacter*), macrolides (*Campylobacter*), virginamycin (enterococci) and avoparcin (enterococci).

Luckily, Vero cytotoxigenic *Escherichia coli* O157, the pathogen responsible for the Wishaw outbreak and other fatalities since, currently shows no antimicrobial resistance in the UK. This probably relates to the fact that in the UK humans suffering from this disease are not treated with antibiotics. Elsewhere in Europe antibiotics are routinely used against this organism and resistant strains do occur.[17]

The other food-borne zoonotic pathogens considered to be of significance are the *Salmonella* spp., still deemed to be responsible for most serious food-poisoning cases. *Salmonella typhimurium* DT104 and other strains of *S. typhimurium* and *S. virchow* have been isolated which are fluoroquinolone-resistant. In addition, 58% of *Salmonella* DT104 isolates are resistant to ampicillin, chloramphenicol, streptomycin, sulphonamides and tetracyclines. The R serotype of this pathogen is additionally resistant to trimethoprim and quinolones, posing a real problem in treatment terms.[18]

There is also evidence that resistance may be transferable from animal to human enterococci, which continue to pose problems in immunocompromised patients. Plasmid-transferred resistance has been demonstrated in two strains isolated in Madagascar of *Yersinia pestis*, the zoonotic causative pathogen of plague, and of considerable concern and significance in terms of world health, especially in the developing world. One strain is streptomycin-resistant – previously the main drug of choice for treating plague – and the other is resistant to chloramphenicol, tetracyclines and sulphonamides – the second-line alternatives.

The WHO believes that there is evidence for arguing that wherever possible, antibiotics should not be extensively used in agriculture, especially where the use is purely to accelerate animal growth to market weight, rather than to treat clinical disease. The emergence of vancomycin-resistant bacteria shows links to the use of the related compound avoparcin, and the introduction of pristinamycin into human therapy has been compromised by use of virginamycin in animal feed.

The WHO has set out a document containing global principles for the containment of antimicrobial resistance in animals intended for food. This suggests that all antimicrobials used for growth promotion should be phased out as soon as possible. Governments are exhorted to refuse or revoke licences for these products. There is also a recommendation that antibiotic use in animals should not be seen as a replacement for good husbandry.[14]

Direct impact of antibiotic resistance on healthcare

This issue is probably of more concern in a secondary care setting where seriously ill patients are treated regularly, and where health policy, especially on prescribing practice, is pioneered. The emergence of MRSA in particular, along with other resistant pathogens in hospital premises, has provoked a measured response with the introduction of antibiotic policies in these establishments. With the move to Primary Care Trusts (PCTs) and the introduction of regional or area formularies, consideration will need to be given to issues of seamless care and antibiotic hierarchies. Coordinated policies for primary and secondary care on antibiotic prescribing could do much to slow the emergence of resistant pathogens.

Antimicrobial resistance in therapy for immunocompromised patients has also become an issue. Regimes for the treatment and continued prophylaxis of the main zoonotic pathogens seen as a threat to these patients must be decided through specialist units with the support of microbiological laboratories and consultants.

In conclusion, there is a need for coordination between not only secondary and primary care, but also animal health specialists to ensure that in the future the therapeutic gains derived from antibiotic use are not lost.

Legislation

A brief mention has been made of the HSE/COSHH regulations previously. As in any other realm of healthcare, practice goes hand in hand with the law. It is almost inevitable that some of these rules and regulations cover aspects of zoonotic diseases. Wherever possible these regulations have been indicated in the sections or chapters relating to the condition caused by the responsible pathogen. The following section assembles some of the more significant measures.

The Health and Safety at Work etc. Act 1974

This act and the statutory instruments and regulations made under it confer a duty of care on employers to ensure that they do not expose their employees to risks in the work place. It requires all employers to draw up a health and safety policy statement, and to provide protective clothing or equipment as required by health and safety law. Likewise, all employees must ensure, as far as possible, their own safety when working.[1]

There is also a requirement to report injuries and certain diseases (including zoonoses) to the HSE. This is covered by the Reporting of Injuries, Diseases and Dangerous Occurrences Regulations (RIDDOR) 1995. These replaced the previous regulations, and came into force in England, Scotland and Wales on 1 April 1996. Under these rules there is a responsibility for an employer or self-employed person to report a case of any disease listed in Schedule 3 of the regulations, once it has been diagnosed in writing by a doctor and when the person concerned is currently employed in an associated work activity.

Zoonotic diseases included in the Schedule include:

- Anthrax
- Avian and ovine chlamydiosis
- Brucellosis
- Leptospirosis
- Lyme disease
- Q fever
- Rabies
- *Streptococcus suis*
- Tetanus
- Tuberculosis

In addition there is a catch-all clause, where any disease that may have stemmed from work activities has to be reported, including those possibly contracted from handling dead bodies or tissues of animals or humans. The section on work-induced lung disease also covers such pathogens as *Chlamydia psittaci*, *Mycobacterium avium* complex and *Cryptococcus neoformans*.

Management of Health and Safety at Work regulations 1992

These regulations are made under the HASAW etc. Act 1974, and require employers to carry out an assessment of the risks in their work place, implement suitable risk control measures and carry out health surveillance on employees. They must also inform employees of any risks in the work place (including zoonoses) and give suitable and adequate training to educate their workers in good practice and prevention measures.

Control of Substances Hazardous to Health regulations 1999

Also made under the HASAW Act 1974 are the COSHH regulations. These classify the pathogens that cause zoonoses as hazardous substances. Under these rules employers and self-employed people are required to assess the risks to health from work activities which involve hazardous substances and prevent or, where this is not reasonably practicable, adequately control exposure to the hazardous substances.

Employers must promote good occupational hygiene, with the emphasis on safe working practices, personal protective equipment and personal hygiene. Safe working practices include avoiding injury from tools or equipment, correct disposal of contaminated sharps, and avoiding other high-risk activities such as handling placental matter or dead animals with the bare hands. Personal protective equipment (PPE) should be used whenever necessary, and must be adequate and appropriate for avoiding infection. The use of gloves, respirators, waterproof aprons, face shields, special overalls or other clothing and footwear when carrying out tasks such as examining animals or assisting at birth is recommended. All PPE should be CE-marked and to the appropriate British standard (BS).

Personal hygiene should be promoted with adequate washing facilities, provision of hot water and soap and a means of drying the hands.

The regulations also lay emphasis on the need for common-sense precautions regarding wound care, first aid, disinfection of animal bedding and housing, mucking out regularly and other precautions which prevent disease transmission. Good husbandry practice of regular worming, prompt vaccination and high standards of care and cleanliness are suggested as appropriate measures to assist disease prevention.

Notifiable disease legislation

There are measures separately enacted that require disease notification for animals, or for humans. As zoonoses affect both categories, the main legislation for both is mentioned below.

Statutory notifications of infectious diseases (human)

The requirement to notify cases of certain infectious diseases first came into force in the late 19th century. Since then the range of diseases has increased and is currently covered by the Public Health (Infectious Diseases) regulations 1988. In Scotland the Public Health (Notification of Infectious Diseases)(Scotland) regulations 1988 require similar notification but also include Lyme disease and toxoplasmosis. In Northern Ireland the equivalent legislation is the Public Health Notifiable Diseases Order (Northern Ireland) 1989.

The system is geared to providing rapid detection of epidemics or mass outbreaks of potentially serious disease. The system is currently administered by the Communicable Disease Surveillance Centre (CDSC), and is known as Notification of Infectious Disease System (NOIDS).

The responsibility for notification rests upon 'the attending medical practitioner', who may range from any doctor in any care setting to the proper officer of the local authority. To gain the speed necessary to prevent epidemics, notification does not rely on clinically proven diagnosis; a presumptive diagnosis is enough, with later confirmation or cancellation.

Under this legislation food poisoning should also be notified. This was defined in respect of the regulations using a DoH definition, which states that food poisoning is 'any disease of an infectious or toxic nature caused by or thought to be caused by the consumption of food or water'.[17]

A wide definition – it does cover all cases, and although it does not permit differentiation between causative organisms, the resulting notification allows some statistical work to take place.

Diseases notifiable under the Public Health (Infectious Diseases) regulations 1988, which are considered to be zoonoses, are (in alphabetic order):

- Acute encephalitis
- Anthrax
- Food poisoning
- Leptospirosis
- Meningitis caused by *Haemophilus influenzae*, or other viruses either specified or unspecified
- Plague
- Rabies
- Relapsing fever
- Tetanus
- Tuberculosis
- Typhus fever
- Viral haemorrhagic fever (i.e. Ebola)
- Viral hepatitis

Note: Because of advances in diagnosis and symptom classification, some of the categories framed at the time of the regulations now include under their general headings conditions which might be caused by zoonotic agents. In those cases the heading has been left open.

Notifiable disease in animals

A variety of measures are in place that require notification of cases of certain infectious diseases in animals. As in human cases, the notification is based on presumption, not necessarily clinical proof, and the diagnosis may be confirmed or cancelled after examination of suitable samples by the Veterinary Laboratory Service.

The applicable legislation is shown in Table 8.3.

Table 8.3 Notifiable disease legislation

Title	Zoonotic diseases covered
Animal Health Act 1981	Anthrax, tuberculosis
Anthrax Order 1991 (under Animal Health Act 1981)	Anthrax
Avian Influenza and Newcastle Disease Order	Influenza, Newcastle disease
Brucellosis Order 1997 (under Animal Health Act 1981)	Brucellosis
Rabies Order 1974 with its various SIs and Schedules	Rabies
Infectious Diseases of Horses Order 1987	Glanders
Specified Disease Order 1996 (under Animal Health Act 1981)	Foot-and-mouth disease, scrapie, *Brucella ovis* (*melitensis*)
Specified Animal Pathogens Order 1998	*Echinococcus multilocularis*, equine morbillivirus, *Trichinella spiralis*
Tuberculosis Orders 1984 (under Animal Health Act 1981)	Tuberculosis
Zoonoses Order 1989, Zoonoses Order 1991 (Northern Ireland)	*Brucella* and *Salmonella* spp.

SIs, Statutory Instruments.

Cases of notifiable diseases must be reported on suspicion to the divisional veterinary manager of DEFRA. The last outbreak or occurrence dates for notifiable zoonoses were anthrax (2001), avian influenza (1992), brucellosis (1993), foot-and-mouth disease (2001), Newcastle disease (1997) and rabies (although the cases did not arise from UK-resident animals: 2001).

Many of the measures relating to notifiable diseases in animals overlap, and relate to previously endemic conditions which are now eradicated or controlled. Others relate to organisms which are classified as emerging, or are seen as posing a significant threat were they to arrive in the UK. Examples are equine morbillivirus (Hendra virus) or *Echinococcus multilocularis*. The last condition is particularly interesting as the Pet Travel Scheme (PETS), otherwise known as pet passports, has specific measures to prevent the introduction of this pathogen (see p. 211).

Points to ponder

To round off this chapter, a few almost random topics relating to medical aspects of zoonoses need consideration.

Choice of companion animal

When individuals choose a pet, they do not routinely consult either a vet or a doctor. In most cases, the decision may be of no consequence whatever. However, where there is a seriously ill or potentially at-risk individual in the equation, either as a sole owner or within a family group, the decision process may be more crucial. The more exotic the pet, the more unusual the range of bacteria and other pathogens it can carry. Reptiles are recognised as carrying unusual strains of *Salmonella*, stray kittens can carry a variety of very interesting pathogens and a bird from a pet shop could be the last straw for an already distressed respiratory patient. The other aspect is that a young animal may be tractable and adorable, but the adult may be less appealing and a lot more difficult.[11]

Guidance as to the suitability of a pet is readily available, usually from veterinary surgeons or groups such as the Pet Health Council. When knowledge is gained that a patient or family is contemplating obtaining a new companion animal, it is essential that they are encouraged to seek the available advice before they take on a creature that could pose a health risk.

Xenotransplantation and transgenic animals

One of the dreams of the late 20th century was the availability of an inexhaustible supply of organs, especially hearts and kidneys, for transplantation from genetically engineered animals. Although still a matter of science future rather than pure science fiction, the realisation of this dream is still probably some years away. The ability of a company to produce Dolly the sheep and Percy the pig was certainly impressive.

The scientific application of cloning technology, with the possibility of manipulating the genetic material of animals to achieve therapeutic breakthroughs, has become more accepted. The existence of transgenic sheep capable of producing human insulin or growth hormone gives hope for many patients and opportunities for profit for drug companies. The use of hearts from transgenic pigs has been suggested as a solution for the chronic shortage of these organs from human donors.[20]

In any of these future initiatives it is necessary to exclude all zoonotic pathogens from the material or organs used. The risks are greater than accidental exposure to the pathogen, as there will be a deliberate introduction of a quantity of animal tissue or material by surgery, or possibly injection.[21]

Following the emergence of variant Creutzfeldt–Jakob disease (vCJD) there is a risk that prion or viral agents could be directly transferred unwittingly from species to species. CJD and scrapie have been induced in unrelated species under laboratory conditions by tissue introduction. Thus, sadly, it appears that turning science fiction into science fact still remains a distant, if not unrealistic dream in this field of endeavour.

Useful addresses

IDIS Ltd World Medicines
Millbank House
171 Ewell Road
Surbiton
Surrey KT6 6AX
Tel: +44 (0)20 8410 0700
e-mail: idis@idis.co.uk.

The Hospital for Tropical Diseases
Mortimer Market
London WC1E 6AU
Tel: +44 (0)20 7387 9300 main switchboard
Tel: +44 (0)20 7388 9600 travel clinic

References

1. Anonymous. *Farmwise HSE 1999*. London: Stationery Office, 2000.
2. Hoff G L, Brawley J, Johnson K. Companion animal issues and the physician. *South Med J* 1999; 92: 651–659.

3. Rodricks J V. Risk assessment, the environment, and public health. *Environ Health Perspect* 1994; 102: 258–264.

4. ILSI Risk Science Institute Pathogen Risk Assessment Working Group. A conceptual framework to assess the risks of human disease following exposure to pathogens. *Risk Anal* 1996; 16: 841–848.

5. Vormbrock J K, Grossberg J M. Cardiovascular effects of human–pet dog interactions. *J Behav Med* 1988; 11: 509–517.

6. Serpell J. Beneficial effects of pet ownership on some aspects of human health and behavior. *J R Soc Med* 1991; 84: 717–720.

7. Wilson C C. The pet as an anxiolytic intervention. *J Nerv Ment Dis* 1991; 179: 482–489.

8. Jewett J F, Hecht F M. Preventive health care of adults with HIV infection. *JAMA* 1993; 269: 1144–1153.

9. Sandouk F, Haffar S, Zada M, *et al.* Pancreatic-biliary ascariasis: experience of 300 cases. *Am J Gastroenterol* 1997; 92: 2264–2267.

10. Spencer L. Study explores health risks and the human animal bond. *J AVMA* 1992; 201: 1669.

11. Grant S, Olsen C W. Preventing zoonotic disease in immunocompromised persons: The role of physicians and veterinarians. *Emerg Infect Dis* 1999; 5. CDC Electronic Journal. http://www.cdc.gov/nicdod/eid/index.htm.

12. Ministry of Agriculture, Fisheries, and Food. *Zoonoses Report UK 1999.* London: HMSO, 1999.

13. Rosenkoetter M M. Health promotion: the influence of pets on life patterns in the home. *Holist Nurs Pract* 1991; 5: 42–51.

14. World Health Organization. *Overcoming Antimicrobial Resistance – World Health Report on Infectious Diseases.* Geneva: WHO, 2000.

15. Report of the House of Lords Select Committee on Science and Technology. *Resisitance to Antibiotics, 3rd Report.* London: House of Lords, March 2001.

16. SMAC (Standing Medical Advisory Committee), Department of Health. *The Path of Least Resistance.* London: HMSO, 1998.

17. Advisory Committee on the Microbiological Safety of Food. *Report on Verocytotoxin-Producing* Escherichia coli. London: HMSO, 1995.

18. Threlfall E J, Ward L R, Rowe B. Increasing incidence of resistance to trimethoprim and ciprofloxacin in epidemic *Salmonella typhimurium* DT104 in England and Wales. *Euro Surveillance* 1997; 2: 81–84.

19. Public Health Laboratory Service. *Statutory Notifications of Infectious Diseases; Notifications of Food Poisoning.* London: PHLS, 2001.

20. Allan J S. Xenotransplantation at a crossroads: prevention vs. progress. *Nature* 1996; 2: 18–21.

21. Michaels M G, Simmons R L. Xenotransplant-associated zoonoses. *Transplantation* 1994; 57: 1–7.

Appendix 1

Web resources

Without access to the literature resources available through the Internet, it is unlikely that this book would ever have been written. The World Wide Web offers the resources of a comprehensive library, with access to a wide range of peer-reviewed scientific papers, at the touch of a keyboard or the click of a mouse.

It is not just technical texts that are available. Many government departments, both at home and abroad, have their own web sites, where information on legislation, statistics and breaking news can be found.

The uniform resource locators (URLs) listed below represent a brief selection of those sites which have been used to assist the research for this publication. The addresses offer the opportunity for students to locate additional information or research topics in depth.

Some of the sites listed require visitors to register before they are able to use all of the facilities. At the time of writing none requires any fee for access. An attempt has been made to arrange the sites in a semblance of order; however, the list is not exclusive or necessarily comprehensive, as new sites appear daily. These sites can offer a jumping-off point for further investigation although, as most people familiar with the 'Net' know, where you start is not always related to where you finish.

European

Council of Europe   http://europa.eu.int/
Institut Pasteur   http://www.pasteur.fr/

International

Food and Agriculture Organization   http://www.fao.org/
  (FAO) of the United Nations
International Association for   hhtp://www.paratuberculosis.org/
  Paratuberculosis
Office International des Epizooties   http://www.oie.int/
  (OIE)
World Health Organization (WHO)   http://www.who.org/

UK

Animal Health Distribution Association (AHDA)	http://www.ahda.org.uk/
Animal Medicines Training Regulatory Association (AMTRA)	http://www.amtra.org.uk/
Association of British Pharmaceutical Industry (ABPI)	http://www.abpi.org.uk/
British Broadcasting Corporation (BBC) news	http://news.bbc.co.uk/
British Equine Veterinary Association (BEVA)	http://www.beva.org.uk/
British Medical Association (BMA)	http://www.bma.org.uk/
British Medical Journal (BMJ)	http://www.bmj.com/
British Small Animal Veterinary Association (BSAVA)	http://www.bsava.com
British Veterinary Association (BVA)	http://www.bva.co.uk/
British Veterinary Poultry Association (BVPA)	http://www.bvpa.freeserve.co.uk/
Chartered Institute for Environmental Health (CIEH)	http://www.cieh.org.uk/
CJD Surveillance Unit	http://www.cjd.ed.ac.uk/
Department of Agriculture and Rural Development (Northern Ireland) (DARDNI)	http://www.dardni.gov.uk/
Department for Environment, Food, and Rural Affairs (DEFRA: *vice* MAFF)	http://maff.gov.uk/defra/
Department of the Environment, Transport and the Regions (DETR)	http://www.detr.gov.uk
Department of Health (DoH)	http://www.open.gov.uk/doh/
Department of Trade and Industry (DTI)	http://www.dti.gov.uk/
Farmers' Weekly	http://www.fwi.co.uk
Food and Drink Federation	http://www.fdf.org.uk/
Food Standards Agency (FSA)	http://www.foodstandards.gov.uk/
Foreign and Commonwealth Office (FCO)	http://www.fco.gov.uk/
Health Education Authority (HEA)	http://www.wiredforhealth.gov.uk/
Health and Safety Executive (HSE)	http://www.hse.gov.uk/
Institute for Animal Health (IAH)	http://www.iah.bbrsc.ac.uk/
Institute of Food Science and Technology (IFST)	http://www.ifst.org/

The Lancet	http://www.thelancet.com/
Meat and Livestock Commission (MLC)	http://www.meatmatters.com/
Medicines Control Agency (MCA)	http://www.open.gov.uk/mca/
Milk Development Council	http://www.mdc.org.uk
Ministry of Agriculture, Fisheries, and Food (MAFF)	http://www.maff.gov.uk/
National Farmers' Union (NFU)	http://nfu.co.uk
National Office of Animal Health (NOAH)	http://www.noah.demon.co.uk
National Pig Association (NPA)	http://www.npa-uk.net/
National Sheep Association (NSA)	http://www.nsa.org.uk/
The People's Dispensary for Sick Animals (PDSA)	http://www.pdsa.org.uk
Pet Food Manufacturers' Association (PFMA)	http://www.pfma.com/
Pet Health Council (PHC)	http://pethealthcouncil.co.uk/
Public Health Laboratory Services (PHLS)	http://www.phls.co.uk/
Royal College of Physicians	http://www.rcplondon.ac.uk/
Royal College of Veterinary Surgeons (RCVS)	http://www.rcvs.org.uk/
Royal Pharmaceutical Society of Great Britain (RPSGB)	http://www.rpsgb.org.uk/
Royal Society for the Prevention of Cruelty to Animals (RSPCA)	http://www.rspca.org.uk
Scottish Environment Protection Agency (SEPA)	http://www.sepa.org.uk/
Scottish Farmers' Weekly	http://www.nfus.org.uk
Society of Practising Veterinary Surgeons (SPVS)	http://www.spvs.org.uk/
Veterinary Laboratory Agency (VLA)	http://maff.gov.uk/aboutmaf/agency/vla
Veterinary Medicine Directorate (VMD)	http://www.vmd.gov.uk/
Veterinary Products Committee	http://www.vpc.gov.uk/

USA

American Veterinary Medical Association (AVMA)	http://avma.org/
Centers for Disease Control and Prevention (CDC)	http://www.cdc.gov/
Center for Food Safety and Applied Nutrition (CFSAN)	http://vm.cfsan.fda.gov/

Department of Agriculture (DoA)	http://www.usda.gov/
Department of Health and Human Services	http://www.hhs.gov/
Food and Drugs Administration (FDA)	http://www.fda.gov/
Medscape	http://www.medscape.com
Nature	http://www.nature.com
New England Journal of Medicine	http://www.nejm.com/
Science	http://www.sciencemag.org/
Scientific American	http://www.sciam.com/

Appendix 2

Case study answers

These are brief answers to the case studies. They are not meant to be exhaustive or extensive. They aim to help consolidate some of the knowledge gained from this book.

Case study 1
1. Yes, it is possible that there is a link between the two.
2. The most likely condition is the respiratory form of psittacosis.
3. Both bird and owner should receive appropriate antibiotic therapy as soon as possible.

Case study 2
1. Unlikely.
2. This woman has a long-standing exposure to cats. It is extremely possible that she could have contracted toxoplasmosis or *Toxocara* at some point in the past and that it has now reactivated due to the steroid therapy, or it could be a fresh infection. Both these pathogens could cause the visual impairment.
3. She should seek medical advice swiftly, and visit an optician. Rapid drastic intervention may be necessary to save her sight.

Case study 3
1. Cutaneous larva migrans.
2. This is usually a self-limiting condition. However, topical tiabendazole (which is not a licensed product in the UK), ivermectin, albendazole or tiabendazole orally have been used.
3. Mr Evans could have helped prevent this by not walking on wet sand barefoot, especially on beaches where dogs had defecated.
4. Probably *Giardia*.
5. The episodic pattern of the condition, and the presence of profound flatulence. Diagnosis is confirmed by isolation of the organism from a stool sample and microscopy.
6. The most likely treatment is a course of metronidazole orally at a dose of 40 mg three times a day for 5 days.

Case study 4

1. Lyme disease.
2. The rash that has appeared around the tick bite, along with the fever and chill symptoms.
3. Either injected benzylpenicillin or a course of oral tetracyclines.
4. Treatment is essential to prevent later complications. The complications, especially in young adults, can be severe, including neurological damage, cardiac damage, and juvenile-onset (Lyme) arthritis.

Case study 5

1. Yes.
2. The likely causative organism is one of the *Cryptosporidium* spp., as these are particularly associated with dogs, and also produce the type of diarrhoea described.
3. The groups of people most at risk from this pathogen are the elderly, immunocompromised patients and young children.
4. Mr Kirkbride will need supportive therapy and nursing to bring him through this attack successfully, with extensive rehydration. He will need to be advised about personal and general hygiene, should consider not having regular contact with the dogs and perhaps even sell the business.

Case study 6

1. No, it is neither safe nor desirable, as there are several zoonotic diseases which would be dangerous to a pregnant woman.
2. The main risk organisms are toxoplasmosis, and *Chlamydia pecorum (psittaci)*. Both can cause neonatal death or disease, and late-term abortion.
3. Mrs McBride should not handle overalls worn by workers that may be contaminated with material from peripartum ewes, or faecal matter.
4. Due to the risk of listeriosis it is advisable that this woman is not involved in cheese-making during her pregnancy, and should not consume any unpasteurised dairy products.

Case study 7

1. Probably not. The advice from Professor Sir Hugh Pennington is that very young children should not go on farm visits as the risks are too great.
2. There is a wide range of risk pathogens for children of this age in this setting, from *Escherichia coli* to *Listeria*, via *Toxocara*, *Cryptosporidium* and *Clostridium perfringens*, just to mention a few.
3. If the farm is to be open to the public, the farmer must ensure that there are adequate hand-washing facilities on site, and a separate area for food consumption.

4.   Educating children not to put their fingers into their mouths after touching animals or soil and faecal material is an essential first step. Encouraging them to wash their hands thoroughly before eating is also important.

Case study 8

1.   Probably anthrax spores, from the imported hides.
2.   Immediate hospitalisation and intensive antibiotic therapy.
3.   As anthrax is notifiable under Reporting of Injuries, Diseases, and Dangerous Occurrences Regulations (RIDDOR), the Public Health (Infectious Diseases) Regulations 1988 or equivalent, and the Anthrax Order 1991, the Health and Safety Executive (HSE), Public Health Laboratory Service (PHLS) and Department for Environment, Food, and Rural Affairs (DEFRA) should all be notified as soon as possible.

Case study 9

1.   The first question should concern his immunisation status. Has he had tetanus vaccination? Is he immunised against rabies? The next question should be to determine the exact time between the bite and his appearance with you.
2.   See a doctor immediately. Initiate rabies immunoglobulin treatment now. Contact the Hospital for Tropical Diseases. Start antibiotic therapy as soon as possible to prevent other infections.
3.   This bite might be non-rabid (we can but hope), but there is also a risk of *Pasteurella* spp., tetanus or other clostridia being present. Make no mistake – this person is in deep trouble.

Index

Page numbers in **bold** refer to major discussions and usually include disease in animals, transmission, disease in humans, diagnosis, treatment and prevention.

Page numbers in *italics* refer to figures and tables.

Entries have been kept to a minimum under 'zoonoses' and readers are advised to seek more specific entries.

All index entries relate to zoonoses, unless otherwise specified.

The following abbreviations have been used as subentries:
AIDS = Acquired Immunodeficiency Syndrome
BSE = Bovine Spongiform Encephalopathy
HIV = Human Immunodeficiency Virus
TSEs = Transmissible Spongiform Encephalopathies
vCJD = variant Creutzfeldt-Jakob disease
WHO = World Health Organization